THE LATINX GUIDE TO LIBERATION

of related interest

Queer Latine Heroes
25 Changemakers from Latin America and the U.S. from History and Today
Sofia Aguilar
Illustrated by Dali Valentino
ISBN 978 1 80501 224 5
eISBN 978 1 80501 223 8

Moving and Identity
Multiculturalism, Somatic Awareness and Embodied Code-Switching®
Marcia Warren
ISBN 978 1 83997 837 1
eISBN 978 1 83997 838 8

Black Creative Healing
Arts-based Approaches to Address Intergenerational and
Race-Based Trauma in African Diasporic Communities
Adenike Webb, PhD, MT-BC and Natasha Thomas, PhD, MT-BC
ISBN 978 1 80501 768 4
eISBN 978 1 80501 769 1

THE LATINX GUIDE TO LIBERATION

Healing from Historical, Generational, and Individual Trauma

VANESSA PEZO

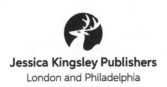

Jessica Kingsley Publishers
London and Philadelphia

First published in Great Britain in 2025 by Jessica Kingsley Publishers
An imprint of John Murray Press

2

Copyright © Vanessa Pezo 2025

The right of Vanessa Pezo to be identified as the Author
of the Work has been asserted by her in accordance with
the Copyright, Designs and Patents Act 1988.

A CIP catalogue record for this title is available from
the British Library and the Library of Congress

ISBN 978 1 80501 021 0
eISBN 978 1 80501 022 7

Printed and bound in Great Britain by Clays Ltd

Jessica Kingsley Publishers' policy is to use papers that are natural,
renewable and recyclable products and made from wood grown in
sustainable forests. The logging and manufacturing processes are expected
to conform to the environmental regulations of the country of origin.

Jessica Kingsley Publishers
Carmelite House
50 Victoria Embankment
London EC4Y 0DZ

www.jkp.com

John Murray Press
Part of Hodder & Stoughton Ltd
An Hachette Company

The authorised representative in the EEA is Hachette Ireland,
8 Castlecourt Centre, Dublin 15, D15 XTP3, Ireland (email: info@hbgi.ie)

This book is dedicated to any of my fellow Latinxs who have ever struggled to feel like they are enough.

This book is also dedicated to the people who made me who I am: Vicenta, Timoteo, Teresa, Adriel, Lupita, Xavier, Bianca, Brianna, Christian, and Abel, and all of my Tías and Tíos.

Contents

Preface 9

A Note on Language: Why "Latinx"? 13

Introduction 17

1. Grasping for the Roots 25

2. The Hidden Truths of Colonialism 38

3. Creating Race in the Americas. 48

4. Making the Invisible Visible 63

5. Soul Wounds 84

6. *La Cultura Cura* 95

7. Immigration Stories Matter 116

8. Twice as Perfect 135

9. Finding Healthy Collectivism 150

10. Freeing Ourselves from the Colonization of Gender . 165

11. Getting Out of Survival Mode and Back into the
    Body. 186

12. Learning to Feel Our Feelings, Challenge Negative Belief Systems, and Process Our Trauma. 210

13. *"Hoy Semillas—Mañana Flores"* (Today Seeds—Tomorrow Flowers) 226

Appendix. 234

References 236

Index 251

Preface

We all come from somewhere, and from someone. For me, my sense of rootedness has always come from the predominantly Mexican community of East Los Angeles, California. More specifically, my *Ama* and *Apa's*[1] house. A house *Apa* moved the family into just after his tenth child, my *Tío* Vicente, was born in the early 1970s. A home where they would raise 12 children in total, and many more grandchildren, myself included.

Apa built this house directly behind the first family home, what we all call "the front house." The front house was where I lived with my parents. Protecting both houses and us from the commotion of the street is a tall wrought iron gate set into concrete. Behind it is a *guayaba* tree, perfect for climbing, offering shade and an additional buffer. These two landmarks of my childhood marked the line we as kids were not allowed to cross alone. On one side of the gate, we had complete freedom, but we all knew never to dare to open or go past the gate alone.

When I was a kid living there in the early 1990s, the street commotion on a good day was the blaring music of the ice-cream truck or the *elotero's* horn. On a bad day it was a drive-by shooting. Some days it was both!

---

1   *Ama* and *Apa* are my maternal grandparents. Everyone in my family, extended family, and beyond, for as long as I can remember, calls them *Ama* and *Apa*. It didn't click for me until I was an adult that *Ama* and *Apa* were Spanish for Mom and Dad, because their presence is something beyond that. *Ama* and *Apa* are sacred.

As a young kid, it never occurred to me that the potential for a shooting was bad, or even that I was in danger. This was just something that happened sometimes. I knew to lie on the ground, wait for the shooting noises to end, and eventually my dad or one of my *tíos* would give the all clear and we could get back to playing. *Ama*, *Apa*, my parents, my *tías*, and *tíos* created such a bubble of security for me and my *primos* that I was never afraid when this happened—an early testament to the fact that it isn't necessarily an event that is traumatic, but what happens to you after the event that matters most.

I had no idea that any type of life aside from the one I was living in my East L.A. neighborhood and school existed until my parents were able to buy a home some 30 miles away in Chino, California. I remember arriving in Chino and finding it so odd that there were no ice-cream trucks, no street vendors. It was so quiet! The only thing filling the air was the odor from the nearby dairy farms owned by Dutch families whose last names seemed to all start with "Van."

When I arrived at my new and mostly white school in second grade as a brown-skinned, brown-eyed girl with silver teeth, I was asked at recess by another kid if I had transferred from "the Mexican" school. Another asked me why I already had braces. This was a clue that silver teeth, practically a rite of passage in East L.A., were not a common occurrence here.

This was my first clue that something was different. For the first time I was different from the kids around me, and these differences were not welcomed. I have been trying to resolve and understand these differences ever since.

Every weekend we went back to East L.A. to spend time with family, to celebrate birthdays and baptisms. Constantly going back and forth between these two communities, these two cultures, these two worlds, made me conscious of racism, classism, stereotypes, and shame long before I had the language to describe them. Language that wouldn't come until much later.

All I knew growing up was that each world pulled me in a different direction and wanted me to be a different version of myself. It was confusing, stressful, and made me feel increasingly insecure. This was acculturative stress, and much of what I was feeling was a normal response to being caught between two cultures. I know this now, but I didn't know it then. Instead, I perceived that I must be wrong in some way.

Always a curious person, I developed a compelling desire to figure out why. I wanted to know why the world was the way it was, and why people were the way they were. I wanted to understand why everything that made me different from the light-skinned, light-eyed, light-haired, solidly middle-class nuclear families I grew up around in Chino was viewed as a deficit.

This desire to understand has been a motivating force in my life ever since. In college I realized that although I am a Latina, Mexican on my mom's side and Ecuadorian on my dad's side, I had never been taught in a formal way about where my family was from, my culture, or our place in society and the world. Latinxs had been strangely absent from the history, literature, and art I had been educated about up to then. I had to seek the knowledge out on my own.

Learning about the history and sociology of Latin America, about culture, and about how modern societies including the U.S. were formed allowed me to look at the world very differently. I saw that so much of what we consider "normal" and measure ourselves against isn't normal at all, it's just whiteness. It has been constructed. It's all about power. The more I came to realize this, the more firmly I could plant my feet as I rejected the lies and degrading stereotypes about Latinx people that have been normalized.

My education has helped me to heal from the experiences I had growing up navigating two different cultures, especially the dominant white culture that sought to exclude and devalue me.

Later, I decided to pursue graduate school at Cal State Long Beach to become a clinical social worker, and eventually a trauma therapist. It was in these early years of my career that all my worlds came together. I saw that the emotional wounds my clients were struggling with were not only the result of their direct experiences of trauma, but the result of generations of experiences, long histories of exclusion and exploitation. They shared stories similar to ones I recognized from my own family.

Many of the traumatic experiences my clients had gone through happened because our oppressive social systems had not only allowed them to happen but had even encouraged them to happen. I saw how patriarchal cultures excused violence against women and children, how racism normalized violence against Black and Brown people and immigrants, how families bore the brunt of brutal capitalism with no safety net.

I came to see again and again that understanding history, culture, and society was paramount to helping those I served to make sense of their experiences and find their version of healing. I saw how their healing rippled outward, and positively influenced those around them like their children and their communities. I developed a strong belief in our innate capacity to heal.

This book is a collection of knowledge I have gained along the way through my education, my formal training, my own healing journey, and in my work of nearly a decade serving my clients as a trauma therapist. This book is my offering to my culture and my community. I am very privileged to have received a quality education, and this book is my way to share what I have learned, so others may benefit from it too.

I hope you find this information to be helpful and even validating. I hope that you can use and apply what you learn here to reinforce your sense of worth and innate value as a sacred member of our culture, to effect positive change on the world around you, for you and others like you, for us. I hope we find collective liberation, *todxs juntxs*, all together.

A Note on Language: Why "Latinx"?

Naming ourselves is important, lest we be named by others.

—PATRICIA ENGEL, FROM "ON NAMING
OURSELVES, OR: WHEN I WAS A SPIC"

"Latinx" is a contentious term in our community. When I've used this word online, I have been told the term Latinx is "just progressives wanting to change everything" and that I should use Latino *only*. I have also been told "I'm not Latinx, I'm Hispanic." Others have said that Latinx is a colonizer term and that we should be calling ourselves Indigenous *only*.[1]

These discrepancies are not surprising considering the Latinx population in the U.S. reached 62.5 million people in 2021. It is hard to fathom that we could get 19% of the entire U.S. population to agree on a singular term to define us. I imagine that in the year 2060 when our numbers are expected to reach 111 million or 28% of the population it might get even harder. We are far from a homogeneous group, and simple and concise concepts won't contain us.

Despite the conflict, I have chosen to use this word to explain the social group of people I belong to and am writing

---

1   For a history on terms that have been used before such as "Hispanic" and "Latino," please see the Appendix.

for. Mainly, because I want it to be clear who this book is for, while being as inclusive as our current language allows.

I use the term Latinx to describe an incredibly diverse social group, and as a label for a constructed social identity— not to subsume any one person's individual identity. Each person can and should define that for themselves.

The origins of the term "Latinx" are unclear. It follows a path like other terms we have seen used by community members before. In the 1960s and 70s, Chicana feminists began to use an "X" in Xicano and Xicana to signify the oppression that Chicanas experienced not only in the U.S., but also within the male-dominated Chicano movement. The "X" was also said to represent a connection to their indigenous roots, which many were rediscovering in this period.

In the 1970s into the 1990s, as global feminism spread, activists in Latin America would X out words ending in -os to reject masculinity as the default identity. In Latin America the "x" has been used by activist groups seeking to create a more inclusive and gender-neutral language. In the early 2000s, Latinx began appearing in Google trends and being used by English-speaking Latinx people in English conversation.

Since the early 2000s, the term Latinx has been on the rise as many see the term as an opportunity to reclaim and redefine identity outside the current patriarchal power structures. Latinx is used to be inclusive of all genders. Latinx moves beyond the binary of the masculine Latino and the feminine Latina.

As "Latinx" grows in popularity its meaning expands. Afroindigenous (Zapotec) poet Dr. Alan Pelaez Lopez has stated:

> the "X" in Latinx is a wound as opposed to a trend that speaks to a collective history. The "X" is attempting to speak to the violences of colonization, slavery, against women and femmes, and the fact that many of us experience such an intense displacement and silence that we have no language in which to articulate who we are.

Latinx came to represent those who have been historically and systematically excluded.

And so, I offer the term Latinx here, not as a redefinition of any one person's identity, but as a term of solidarity. I use Latinx with the understanding that the Latinx community is multinational, multiethnic, multilingual, and multiracial. I use Latinx in recognition of the many differences between individuals within the group including race, ethnicity, disability, class, gender, sexuality, immigration status, and citizenship type, and in recognition of how these differences shape lived experiences. Latinx represents a myriad of socio-political identities while acknowledging the history of colonialism that brought us all together. Latinx represents a group of people with a vision of community, solidarity, healing, and liberation from oppression of all kinds.

One day we may move beyond Latinx, as our community grows, and as the socio-political structures around us evolve. Language, like identity, is fluid and can change over time. I choose to use Latinx now allowing the X to also signify the intersection of multiple identities, multiple peoples, and to represent this moment and place in time. I look forward to the day when liberation from oppression allows us to not only imagine but to embody the identities that most feel like home.

INTRODUCTION

BEGINNING THE PROCESS

The beginning of any healing process can be daunting. It is a commitment to confront a wound and then take the steps necessary to allow it to begin healing. Sometimes in the process of healing, things hurt more before they start to feel better. And healing from the wounds of trauma, oppression, and colonization is no different.

When I begin working with a new client, we always start with a conversation about how we're going to address their current concerns to find healing. I often give a similar version of this statement:

> I am a trauma therapist. That doesn't necessarily mean we are going to be talking about trauma in detail every time we meet. What it does mean is that trauma is the lens I look through as I try to understand and help you. A lot of the distress or problems we struggle with today have been shaped by our past experiences. And when we can look at a present-day problem or issue or behavior or "symptom," and trace it back to where it started, it often makes a lot more sense. As we shift our view away from "what is wrong with me?" and towards "where did this start and why did this start?" you'll have more insight into yourself, and your reactions, and with that deeper understanding comes more power to make change.

What works with my clients on a one-to-one level can also be expanded outward and applied to how we heal our families and our culture. If we can reach the source, the root of our pain, we can apply medicine to this wound. We can give gentle care and attention to the place where the suffering comes from, and we can let go of the blame or shame that comes from focusing only on our problems. When we better understand, we can heal.

DEFINING TERMS
Trauma
According to the Substance Abuse and Mental Health Services Administration (SAMHSA):

> trauma results from an event, series of events, or set of circumstances that is experienced by an individual as physically or emotionally harmful or threatening and that has lasting adverse effects on the individual's functioning and physical, social, emotional, or spiritual well-being... Traumas can affect individuals, families, groups, communities, specific cultures, and generations.

Historical trauma
Historical trauma describes the responses to massive violence and subjugation experienced by a collective group. Lakota social work researcher Maria Yellow Horse Brave Heart, PhD explains that historical trauma is "cumulative emotional and psychological wounding across generations, including the lifespan." Public health researcher Michelle Sotero, PhD notes that historical trauma isn't the result of one single violent event but violence over an extended period as one dominant population deliberately targets and subjugates another.

Historical trauma in the Latinx community includes the genocide and displacement of our Indigenous ancestors, the enslavement of our African ancestors, and the subsequent racism, sexism, discrimination, economic oppression, political violence, and xenophobia we have been subjected to in the world that colonialism created at our expense.

Generational trauma

Generational trauma refers to how traumatic stress and survival responses are passed down within a family or a culture from one generation to the next. When one generation survives trauma such as civil war, forced migration, discrimination, familial abuse, and violence, the traumatic stress reactions, survival adaptations, and resiliency strategies they develop can be passed to the next generations.

Epigenetic science gives us some clues on how trauma is passed on. Research, such as that by Professor of Psychiatry Rachel Yehuda, PhD and colleagues, suggests that trauma and stressful environments can alter the functional expression of our genes. Offspring can then inherit these epigenetic modifications resulting in the transmission of traumatic stress reactions. These changes can affect how subsequent generations experience stress and increase susceptibility to mental health conditions and other adverse reactions. Research by Dr. Yehuda has found that parental trauma exposure is associated with greater risk for post-traumatic stress disorder in the next generation.

Trauma can also be passed through nurture and caregiving practices. Trauma can influence the way parents interact with and respond to the needs of their children. Trauma survivors may develop reactions such as increased fear, avoidance, and a negative view of themselves, others, and the world. These emotional responses and beliefs impact the way some survivors of trauma parent. Children model their behavior and expectations of others after their experiences with parents and caregivers. When a parent's orientation to the world is one of being under threat, children may absorb and display some of these responses.

Trauma can also be passed via cultural practices and rituals that transfer historical knowledge across generations. Vamik Volkan in "Transgenerational transmissions and chosen traumas" explains that the shared experience of trauma can become one component of a large group's identity as it is an experience that brings them all together while differentiating them from others. The survival of collective trauma influences the story the community tells about the world, about itself, and about its survival. Each generation will learn and make new meaning of this story.

Individual trauma

Individual trauma refers to a person's lived experience of trauma and its effects, which can include a variety of mental, emotional, cognitive, physical, and spiritual reactions and alterations. These reactions can stem from a person's experience of dangerous or overwhelming life events, or from chronic circumstances such as living within an abusive environment or oppressive society. These reactions may also be shaped by generational and historical sources of trauma.

Liberation

This is the freedom of humanity from systems of colonialism, exploitation, hierarchy, violence, and oppression that perpetuate great harm to bring about a world where all living beings can live in collective harmony together with mother earth. The path to liberation begins with the development of critical consciousness, learning to see and question the oppressive nature of social, political, and economic structures.

CONFUSING TRAUMA FOR CULTURE

Sadly, I have heard my fellow Latino/a/xs at times refer to "Toxic Latino" culture as the root of many problems for our community. However, what is being perceived as negative qualities of our culture are signs of historical or generational trauma that can be healed.

Trauma specialist and somatic abolitionist Resmaa Menakem, in his book *My Grandmother's Hands*, says:

> After months or years, unhealed trauma can appear to become part of someone's personality. Over even longer periods of time, as it is passed on and gets compounded through other bodies

in a household, it can become a family norm. And if it gets transmitted and compounded through multiple families and generations, it can start to look like culture. But it isn't culture. It's a traumatic retention that has lost its context over time.

Looking at ourselves and our culture through the lens of unhealed trauma, we see clearly that culture isn't the problem. Culture has largely been a resource for survival. However, some of the adaptations we have made to survive have been harmful. We adapted first to survive the brutality of the conquest, then to live under colonization, and now to exist in a world of neo-colonization, cultural imperialism, and white supremacy. Pain has rippled through bodies, and families over generations. Responses to that pain now look like culture.

La cultura has been formed through determination and struggle. We have not only survived, we have thrived in community, and maintained many of our pre-colonial values and practices. At times, however, we have been bruised under the weight of extreme violence and domination – and perhaps, we don't need some of those harmful adaptations anymore. Perhaps we can begin to be liberated from this suffering and begin to imagine ourselves and our community beyond it. Perhaps we can rid ourselves, our families, our communities, our culture of the toxic infection of the imposed colonial mindset and worldview that causes us harm.

GOING THROUGH THIS BOOK

In this book, we will explore together how systems of power and domination rooted in colonialism and significant historical events have created historical, generational, and individual trauma for the Latinx people.

Latinx psychology—our mental and emotional characteristics, attitudes, values, behaviors, and worldviews—cannot be understood without viewing them within the context of history. History influenced the way our Latinx identities and psychology have developed.

Pioneer Latinx psychologist Manuel Ramírez III PhD explains in *The Handbook of Chicana/o Psychology and Mental Health* (Velásquez *et al.* 2004) that "the person is an open system...the person is inseparable from the physical and social environments in which he or she lives." Dr. Ramírez explains that as Latinx people we are influenced by the environments we live in, and we also influence those environments. History and time are considered one of these environments. Latinx psychology honors the person-in-environment view, and our complex interconnected relationship to the world around us.

Each of the circles below represents a physical and social environment. Another way of viewing this is that each circle is a context within which we live our lives. Each environment influences and is influenced by the others. When a person's individual characteristics are well suited to their environments, they will experience optimal health and wellness. When there are conflicts between the environments or the person's qualities do not fit the preferences of the environment, they will experience negative outcomes such as vulnerability to trauma, poor mental health, and challenges meeting their goals.

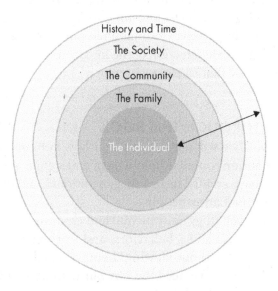

Figure I.1: Person-in-Environment Perspective

In the following chapters we will explore these environments from the outside and move our way in, because history and time are the context within which everything else happens. We will begin with significant historical events that have shaped the Latinx identity, historical trauma, and the formation of oppressive social structures, including white supremacy culture. At a community level we will honor the strengths and healing resources our culture offers to us and explore some common issues Latinx people face, such as immigration and navigating between different cultural expectations. Lastly, we will explore the individual experience, and how our experiences of trauma may manifest in our minds and bodies. We will end with our radical vision for the future.

In each chapter we will use reflection and deconstruction questions to engage in "praxis," a term coined by Brazilian educator Paulo Freire in the book *Pedagogy of the Oppressed* to mean "reflection and action upon the world in order to transform it."

Praxis is a practice central to liberation. Praxis develops our critical consciousness. When we are critical of the social, political, and economic systems that create collective trauma and oppress, we find avenues for action towards our goal—liberation for all oppressed people and an end to cycles of trauma that burden those who have been oppressed. As we grow in our consciousness about the reality of the world, we can build from this new understanding paths towards transformative action and transformative healing.

Reflection and deconstruction questions will also allow us to question the way systems of power and domination have influenced our minds, altering perception of ourselves, others, and the world.

We will evaluate what we've been taught by the dominant culture, challenge harmful narratives, and create new forms of knowledge and understanding for ourselves. We will unlearn to relearn, while anchoring into our cultural strengths and ancestral wisdom. We will draft new narratives, write our own reality, and engage in practices of transformational healing.

I encourage you to use a journal as a safe container for your process as you read this book. Allow yourself space and time for reflection as well as time to integrate. If things begin to feel too much or overwhelming, you can always return to the breath.

Reflection and deconstruction

★ What does liberation mean to you?

CHAPTER 1

GRASPING FOR THE ROOTS

Civilizations Disrupted

CIVILIZATIONS DISRUPTED

El que no sabe es como el que no ve (He who doesn't know is like he who doesn't see) (Spanish proverb)

RESPIRACIÓN PROFUNDA (DEEP BREATH)

As we begin this journey, there may be times when the material becomes overwhelming, triggering, spiritually or even physically painful. This is a normal and natural response to this work, and to learning about the experiences of our ancestors. It is okay. *Estás bien.* And there is nothing wrong with you. There is nothing wrong with feeling deeply. I encourage you to take breaks as often as you need, allowing yourself the space and time to engage with the reflection questions, to write, and to integrate what you are taking in.

Prior to beginning the next section, let us ground and connect inward. And if at any point later while reading you need a break or a pause, return to this practice and allow yourself to be gently guided back into the present.

First, I invite you to begin by allowing your body to settle in wherever you are—maybe you are sitting in a chair or lying down, but wherever you are, take a moment to shift or move anything you need to allow yourself to be just a little more comfortable.

Next, notice what it feels like as your body is gently supported by whatever holds you now—maybe you are seated in a sturdy chair, or on a soft couch, maybe you're touching something soft, or something firm, maybe your feet are planted on the ground. Just notice what it feels like to be held here, gently supported, in this moment...

And then, when you are ready, take a moment to notice your breath...notice the nice gentle *inhale*...and the *exhale*... connecting to the rhythm of your own breathing for just a moment or two.

When you are ready, begin to breathe in gently through the nose for a count of three seconds, and at the top of the inhale pause for a moment holding that breath, then exhale slowly out of the mouth for a count of seven seconds (whoosh). And again, breathe gently in through the nose for three, pause and hold, and then nice and slow out of the mouth for seven (whoosh). Let the exhale be as long and slow as you can get it.

Allow yourself to find a soft rhythm. Maybe noticing how your belly rises, and falls, as you breathe here gently for a few cycles of breath. And when you're ready, as you end, press your feet firmly into the floor if you can, or press your body against whatever holds you now, and feel the presence of this moment. Allow a few muscles to tense tightly, and then softly relax, maybe tensing your hands into fists and then relaxing them, maybe your calves tighten and soften, or your thighs... Let them tense for a few seconds before releasing into relaxation.

Feel yourself here, and now. And whenever you need to, I invite you to return to this place, to this practice, and to your body.

CIVILIZATIONS DISRUPTED

In the story of Latin America and the Caribbean it often seems as if the history of these regions begins at the conquest; as if the arrival of Europeans on ships sparked the commencement of history in a place without its own. While it is true that the concepts of a Latin America or a Caribbean didn't exist yet, something much greater did, and the new arrivals went to great lengths to destroy its existence.

The erasure of Indigenous peoples' history, knowledge, and symbolism from the pre-colonial era happened quite literally. The Europeans burned Indigenous books, records, art, and images. Famously, Spanish bishop Diego de Landa ordered that Mayan codices be burned. Among other things, these codices held religious texts, property records, village and family records, agricultural knowledge, and calendars. The invaders tore down sacred temples throughout Latin America and erected Catholic churches on top of their remains. They used the stones from the dismantled temples to construct their churches as a way of expressing their dominance and disrespect for all that had existed before. They tried to eradicate entire groups of people, and their accomplishments. But what they didn't realize is those people, who they deemed so insignificant, were as much a part of those places as the land, the water, the trees, and the sun. And they could not be disappeared.

What makes our history so dangerous to the colonizers, and those who hold power now, is that it provides us with other models for civilization. There are other ways of organizing human life, and other ways of making sense of our place on this earth. Looking back, we are reminded that we exist as people with an important cultural heritage separate from our relationship to the colonizer. We are not defined by the labels or narratives placed on us by colonialism. We once lived in communities based on mutual care and an intimate connection to the earth and all of creation, and can again. It is easy to see why the colonial powers that be might find Gloria Anzaldua's statement of "This land was Mexican once, was Indian always and is. And will be again" quite threatening.

When the Europeans arrived, they didn't realize or perhaps didn't care that they were interrupting the natural trajectory of advanced societies that had thrived there for thousands upon thousands of years. Mesoamerican civilization was developed in Mexico and Central America. Societies such as the Olmec, Zapotec, Maya, Toltec, and Mexica flourished at different points during this era. Andean civilization developed in the areas now known as Ecuador, Bolivia, Peru, Chile, and Argentina. Groups including the Quechua, Aymara, and Inka were prominent at different points in Andean history.

Both the Mesoamerican and Andean civilizations accomplished incredible feats in architecture, agriculture, social organization, mathematics, and astronomy. A full history of the development and accomplishments of these highly advanced civilizations is beyond the scope of this book, but one point that is key to explore is their worldview, called cosmovision. Mesoamerican and Andean cosmovision shows us that another way of structuring and perceiving the world is possible. Within their cosmovision we may find seeds to be planted and sown within as we conceptualize our own liberated futures.

Both the Mesoamerican and Andean civilizations saw human beings as existing in sacred unity with the natural world and a cosmic order. The nature of reality is that everything is sacred and interconnected. Life was controlled by unseen powers that were all encompassing. Mesoamerican and Andean worlds were designed to reflect this cosmovision.

In Mesoamerican and Andean civilizations, all interactions and ways of life were understood through cosmovision. Ceremonies and rituals were a symbolic expression of human participation in the universe and connection to all other sacred beings. Rituals preceded action to gain the favor of the supernatural or to keep the gods satisfied. All actions, big or small, had religious significance as an experience of the energy connection with the earth and universe.

Existence was intertwined with land, livelihood, and the greater forces of the universe. Land was a living being, sacred, and responsive to human behavior. Land was seen as the home of the ancestors and as a conscious being. Land was held communally. The people and the territory were inseparable as the group's very definition included its relation to the common territory and its history. Spirituality was imbued in all aspects of life, and every act had sacred meaning and function. Work represented a harmonious relationship with the natural world, so it had not only an economic function, but also a social and religious one.

In both Mesoamerican and Andean civilizations, the core unit of society was the family or kinship groups who shared a collective territory. In the Andes, these were called *ayllus*. Together they farmed their shared lands, and worked to raise animals, hunt, gather, weave, and create. Extended networks of *ayllus* would come together for larger projects such as harvesting, building a home, performing a ceremony, or for celebrations, which were frequent.

The diverse activities of the community brought security to Indigenous communities. They could be self-sufficient and meet all of their needs within their local community networks. Cooperation within the community was based on reciprocity, participation, and obligation. Everyone helped each other, knowing that when it was their turn, they would also receive help. Everyone participated.

Cooperation and mutual aid were not only limited to family groups. Rulers used draft systems to complete public works projects, such as building roads, public buildings, or military service. The Inka, who were in power at the time of the European arrival, called this the *mita*. This term was later adopted by the Spanish. Workers were compensated fully for their labor, receiving food or other goods. Rulers, who received tribute such as food or cloth, would also redistribute these goods when needed, such as during a time of famine or war. Because these societies formed around values of cooperation and participation, accumulation of wealth or resources was seen as negative. Full individual development and prestige were earned through community service, not the accumulation of personal wealth. Participation was rewarded with group membership and belonging. This social system was designed to support and reinforce core basic human needs of safety, belonging, self-worth, community actualization, and cultural progression.

It can be difficult for us to fully imagine large societies structured this way, people interacting in this way, and the reverence with which our ancestors approached daily living, because this requires a completely different model of reality than most of us live within. Our current society is controlled by a hugely different set of values that bleed into every institution we interact with. Indigenous groups throughout Latin America and the Caribbean have worked to preserve their cultural heritage and ways of life, making it difficult for colonialists to completely erase what was. In later chapters, we will explore the values of our current Western society, and the impact they have on our mindsets and emotions. We will also explore ways we have maintained Mesoamerican and Andean influence within the Latinx culture.

THE ARRIVAL

History does not start with the ingress of the Europeans, but it does represent a major turning point in the evolution and survival of Indigenous peoples in the Americas and the Caribbean. In 1492, Columbus arrived to what is now the Bahamas, seeking gold, silver, pearls, salt, spices, and whatever other exotic treasures could be extracted for Spain. His hope was that he would come upon the treasures Marco Polo had written about by developing a new trade route with Asia.[1]

Columbus' voyage was financed by Spanish monarchs Isabella I of Castille and Ferdinand II of Aragon, who approached this expansion into new territories with a religious zeal. They were encouraged by their recent victory in the reconquest of

---

1   Columbus thought he had arrived in modern day Japan, and he died still believing he had arrived in Asia. In homage to his confusion, in 2020 comedian Ziwe tweeted "throw every christopher columbus statue in the ocean and let that dizzy bitch think he discovered Atlantis."

the Iberian Peninsula.[2] The kingdom of Spain had previously engaged in a centuries-long religious war against the Moors to regain control over the Iberian Peninsula. The Moors were Muslim and originally from Northern Africa. Spain's goal was to ensure the Iberian Peninsula would be Catholic. They accomplished their goal, also in 1492, by winning a final war in Granada and bringing the region fully under Christian control.

At the time of arrival, the Spanish mentality towards expansion into new lands was already deeply intertwined with the expansion of Christianity. They used religion to justify what would follow in the place they called the "New World." When Pope Alexander VI, a fellow Spaniard, ordained Queen Isabella the master of the New World, the blessing by the church of the conquest and colonization was complete.

The Portuguese were not far behind. They had also fought against the Moors in the Iberian Peninsula, but their reconquest ended in the mid-1200s when they took control of most of the western coast. Their focus in the interim had been expansion into Africa. By the 1400s, Portuguese ships were carrying goods back into European markets. In the year 1500, the first Portuguese fleet arrived to what is now Brazil, led by Pedro Alvares Cabral. Like Columbus, he too had intended to go to India, and arrived here by mistake (unlike Columbus, he continued and did eventually get to India).

At first, the land that would come to be known as Brazil was of little interest to the Portuguese. They were preoccupied by their other trade routes that connected them to Africa and Asia. The Portuguese had recently established the transatlantic slave trade, which would become the largest forced movement of people in history. Unfortunately, this plays a pivotal role later during colonization. It was only when French ships arrived at the coast of Brazil in the 1530s that the king of

---

2   The Iberian Peninsula is the southern tip of Europe shared by Spain and Portugal. The peninsula sits right above Africa, separated by the narrow Strait of Gibraltar, which was crossed in both directions by different groups for both migration and invasion.

Portugal began to send Portuguese settlers to Brazil to protect his claim to the land and those who lived on it.

SOCIETIES AT THE TIME OF ARRIVAL

At the time of arrival there were distinct societies who were prominent in Mesoamerica, the Andes, and the Caribbean. It would be them who faced the strange people who arrived on ships. Dominant in Mesoamerica were the Mexica people in the central valley of modern-day Mexico, often referred to as the Aztec Empire. Their capital city Tenochtitlán was a thriving cultural center and the largest and most powerful city in Mesoamerica. The Mexica's incredible achievements included advanced agricultural practices utilizing *chinampas* or floating gardens, mandatory education for all, regardless of gender or class, and a public health and sanitation system more advanced than any other city that existed at that time (yes, including in Europe!).

The Maya, also Mesoamerican, lived in the areas now known as southern Mexico, Guatemala, Belize, and parts of Honduras and El Salvador. The Maya were previously one of the most advanced civilizations of the era but had experienced a decline before the Spanish arrived. The Maya made great advances in architecture. They built pyramids, monuments, and temples that can still be visited today. They developed a sophisticated writing system, were skilled astronomers, creating an accurate calendar and recording lunar and solar cycles. The Maya may have also been the first to discover the concept of zero.

In the Andes of South America, the Inka empire covered modern day Peru, Ecuador, eastern and south-central Bolivia, northwest Argentina, and parts of Chile and Colombia. The Inka connected their empire with an advanced 14,000-mile road system, some of which is still in use today. The Inka population peaked at 10 million. It was the largest and wealthiest empire of the pre-Hispanic period, and at the time of European arrival it was the largest nation in the world.

Inhabiting the islands of the Caribbean were several eth-nically diverse groups, including the Caribs (also known as the *Kalinago*) and the largest group the Tainos (also known as the *Arawaks*). The Taino society was divided into different kingdoms that used a matrilineal descent system and included women as chiefs. They were adept at water travel, building canoes that could hold up to 100 people. They taught their his-tory to younger generations using songs and had complex rit-uals and ceremonies to honor their gods and life's transitions.

In Brazil, the Portuguese encountered a variety of semi-no-madic forest-dwelling groups, including the Tupi, who were tropical rainforest farmers, fishermen, and hunters. Although it is difficult to be certain, estimates state that there were hun-dreds of tribes totaling a population of about three million living in modern-day Brazil when the Portuguese fleet first landed.

THE CONQUEST

In the conquest of the New World, the Spanish first focused on the Caribbean. Columbus quickly set out on a hunt for gold. When the Arawaks, who Columbus described as "the best people in the world," couldn't produce the amount he expected, he directed a military campaign against them, cap-turing 1500 and sending 500 to be sold in the slave markets of Seville.

In 1495, Columbus created a tribute system requiring all males over the age of 13 to produce a hawk's bell full of gold every three months or have their hand cut off. This quota was nearly impossible. The Arawaks resisted by digging up their own cassava crops, and destroying supplies, hoping a famine would force out the Spaniards. Later, they took great pains to avoid having children, and even completed suicides to save future generations from enduring the fate of forced labor and Christianity under tortuous conditions. The Arawaks had a population of at least 100,000 in 1492. By 1542, only 200 were left.

Meanwhile, the Portuguese struggled in their conquest of Brazil. Their goal was to export sugar, a high value crop, back to Europe. Sugar was attractive because it is easy to transport and could not be grown in Europe. To begin establishing sugar plantations they needed to clear land, plant and harvest the crop, and then prepare the sugar to be shipped and sold. Sugar requires a lot of labor, and the Portuguese looked to the local population for their labor supply.

The Portuguese struggled to settle two thousand miles of coastal land. The king began to hand out parcels to wealthy "captains" who could attempt to establish settlements and rule on his behalf. As these captains failed and Indigenous groups destroyed settlements, the king increased Portuguese presence by assigning a royal governor and building a capital city. The Portuguese efforts to capture and enslave people like the Tupi, and the creation of settlements, led to the near extinction of the native populations. The Tupi gradually disappeared as a distinct group. They died from war and disease, were pushed deeper into the forest, or intermixed with the Portuguese.

After the Caribbean, the Spanish moved into Mexico and South and Central America. Some of the conquest was funded by the crown, and others financed their own voyages, the rule being that one-fifth of everything went back to the crown. Everyone was after wealth and riches, but they justified their missions as Christian expansion. When the conquistadors arrived to advanced cities like Tenochtitlán they sought gold and silver with an unquenchable thirst. Indigenous informants, quoted by Miguel Leon-Portilla in *The Broken Spears: The Aztec Account of the Conquest of Mexico*, later described their impressions of the Spanish as they were presented with gifts on arrival. Indigenous informants said they smiled when they saw gold: "They longed and lusted for gold... They hungered like pigs for the gold." They also noted "The strangers' bodies are completely covered...their skin is white as if it were made of lime."

One of the significant advantages for the Europeans was that due to their place in the Iberian Peninsula, the Spanish and Portuguese were accustomed to encountering people of different ethnicities, cultures, and religions. The Indigenous populations, however, had no prior experience to help them understand such strange people who arrived suddenly and looked and behaved so differently. They had never seen Europeans or Africans before. They could never have imagined their motivations, their view of the world as a place for the taking, and their lust for gold and silver. They could have never fathomed what these strange people were willing to do in the pursuit of their goals.

During the conquest, the Spanish conquistadors used superior weaponry like steel blades, crossbows, canons, muskets, and pistols. Their weapons terrorized the Indigenous populations, who had never seen arms so deadly. The weapons were powered by explosive fiery gunpowder, which startled and scared them, again as it was something they had not seen before. The Spanish also used attack dogs and fought on horseback. Horses at that point were extinct in Latin America, and chief Tecum, a Mayan leader, once beheaded the horse of Pedro de Alvarado believing it was a part of the conquistador's own body.

The conquistadors were masters of manipulation. They exploited pre-existing divisions and grievances to weaken the power of Montezuma, leader of the Mexica (Aztec) Empire. They formed alliances with rival groups who resented the Mexica's power over the region. These allies provided support to the Spanish in their conquest. The Spanish also exploited a split in the Inka empire between brothers Huáscar and Atahualpa, who were engaged in a civil war to become *Sapa Inka* (emperor). Diseases brought by the Spanish spread via trade routes, and ravaged the Inka ruling family, pitting the two brothers against each other, and distracting from the Spanish arrival.

The Spanish, knowing they were greatly outnumbered, often relied on grand shows of violence and mayhem to shock the natives, and beat them down not only physically but psychologically. Their goal was to kill as many as possible, which contrasted the Indigenous peoples' style of battle where warriors often focused on taking captives. Described in *The Broken Spears*, Hernán Cortés and his men were once invited to the festival of Toxcátl. Just as the Dance of the Serpent began, as warriors hoped to show the Spanish the beauty of their rituals, and the crowd was shouting "Show us how brave you are! Dance with all your hearts!" the Spanish began to block all the entrances. They trapped and then ambushed the jovial festival goers, slaughtering the celebrants.

Pizarro, inspired by what Cortes had done to Montezuma, used a similar strategy to ambush Atahualpa and his army. Pizarro invited Atahualpa to meet in a square where the Spanish had hidden cannons; 168 Spaniards fired cannons onto thousands of Inka warriors, and then charged in on horseback armed with swords. They slaughtered thousands, and Atahualpa was taken hostage. Atahualpa, sensing the greed of his captors, offered to fill a room with gold in exchange for his release. Pizarro accepted the offer. Atahualpa's people brought a total of 24 tons of gold and silver, the largest ransom in history. After receiving the ransom, Pizarro didn't keep his word and ordered Atahualpa to be burned to death. Atahualpa died by strangulation, a final act of mercy granted in exchange for his conversion to Christianity just before his execution.

As the Europeans hunted riches, their physical bodies became the most effective weapon against the native populations of the Americas and Caribbean—one of infection and contamination. The Spanish and Portuguese infected the Indigenous peoples with bacterial and viral infections they had no immunity to. Deadly diseases like smallpox, typhus, measles, and yellow fever spread rapidly through Indigenous populations, killing them by the millions. Pandemics and epidemics would repeatedly attack Indigenous populations through the 17th and 18th centuries. As millions died of disease, and cities were taken with violence, the empires and lands of the Americas and Caribbean came under the fist of Spanish and Portuguese control. In 1521, Tenochtitlán fell, and the Mexica Empire collapsed, to be followed in 1533 by

Cuzco and the Inka Empire. In 1548, the Portuguese appointed a governor and built the capital city Salvador.

The exact population of the Americas and Caribbean prior to the conquest is difficult to establish. John Kicza, in *The Indian in Latin American History*, writes that there were almost 75 million people in the Americas and Caribbean in 1492. Geographer Alexander Koch and colleagues estimate that European arrival in 1492 led to 56 million deaths by 1600. The Native people of the Americas were killed in massive numbers, while those native to the Caribbean were practically exterminated. These people were scientists, artisans, builders, astronomers, hunters, gatherers, farmers, warriors, priests, mathematicians, healers, teachers, mothers, and fathers. These were complex, beautiful, spiritual, passionate, intelligent, and creative human beings. They lived in groups and societies quite different from the ones most of us live in today. And as the plague from Europe arrived, they were decimated, and much of their humanity was forcibly extinguished. One century and a half later it is estimated that 3.5 million natives were left. A genocide had occurred unlike any that had ever been seen before and will, it is hoped, never be seen again.

If at this point or at any time during your reading you notice a weight on your chest, rapid breathing, tension in your muscles, a sense of disconnection, or any distress, return to our breathing exercise before going on.

CHAPTER 2

THE HIDDEN TRUTHS OF COLONIALISM

On the path to trauma healing, we face the roots of our present-day issues and challenges—not only to name and bear witness to what has happened, but to also revisit the narratives that have formed about these events. It is often those in power who get to write the stories and shape the discourse.

Healing means reclaiming our ability to tell our stories. When we write history, we can shine light on what has been hidden or denied. The dominant historical narrative has diminished the genocide of Indigenous peoples, the enslavement of Africans, and the plunder of Latin American wealth as if these are modest acts. History holds up Europe as a beacon for progress and civilization, not because of its superiority, but because history is written from its perspective. It becomes incredibly important for Latinx people to discover what has been minimized or hidden away. We become more powerful actors in this world through the reclaiming of knowledge of all types.

COLONIZATION

The horrific conquest was only the beginning of the Spanish and Portuguese presence in what is now Latin America and the Caribbean. They would go to extreme ends in their pursuit of draining every last bit of wealth from the New World.

The Europeans' next step was to establish colonies giving them control over lands and control over people. While Brazil attempted to enslave the native populations and force them to work, the Spanish, because they were low in numbers and faced much larger Native populations, chose to take over already established systems of tribute. In Mesoamerica and the Andes, people were already accustomed to providing agricultural surplus and labor to Native rulers; however, these systems would be drastically changed.

The Spanish implemented the *encomienda* system. The *encomienda*, the literal translation being "to entrust," was an estate granted by the crown to the Spanish conquistadors and early settlers. Not only did the new *encomendero*, the owner, get the land, he also got the people on it. The Indigenous people were "entrusted" to the *encomendero*. They now owed him tribute, usually paid with labor but later this included goods and eventually cash payments. The Spanish justified this labor exploitation as a religious mission via the "gift" of Christianity. Catholic priests were also a colonial presence on the *encomiendas* as the Catholic church also sought to grow its power in the colonies. *Encomiendas* were sites of extreme exploitation and abuse.

The *encomenderos* became a noble class, living off the labor of the Native farmers. In the 1570s, the Spanish implemented the *mita*. The *mita* was a system of forced labor which required Indigenous communities to provide one seventh of their male labor force for agriculture, mining, textile factories, and more. These systems of control, the *encomienda* and the *mita*, had consequences beyond the organization of land and labor. They were expressions of dominance and control. The Europeans destroyed the local family structures, changed agricultural production to focus on cash crops, which forced the natives to abandon sustainable farming practices they had used for centuries, all while the population continued to struggle due to rampant disease.

The colonial economies that developed in Latin America had one sole purpose—to enrich the colonizer to the maximum amount possible. For the Spanish empire, silver would become the foundation. In areas like Potosí in what is now Bolivia, and in Zacatecas and Guanajuato of Mexico, there was a silver rush and Natives were fed to the mines in exchange for silver. Seven out of ten taken to the mines never returned.

Indigenous peoples, including women and children, were taken from their agricultural communities and forced to work the mines. Here they struggled under horrific working conditions. Toxic mercury was used to extract the silver, which poisoned the workers. The workers inhaled toxic fumes, causing their hair and teeth to fall out. The Indigenous laborers carried the metal out on their backs. They were injured frequently and often sick, as they moved between the sweltering heat of the mines to the freezing outdoors. In places like Potosí, the mine was on the *cerro rico*, rich mountain, at over 15,000-foot elevation. To keep the laborers working, they were fed pain- and hunger-killing coca leaves. During the colonial period, over eight million Inka miners died in just the Viceroyalty of Peru.

The Spanish were not the only ones searching for precious metals in the mountains. In 1692, Brazil, which had mostly focused on cash crops like sugar and tobacco up to this point, had its own gold rush in Minas Gerais. By 1720, diamonds were discovered as well. Any time resources were discovered the Indigenous people of that place were either killed, expelled, or forced to supply labor.

Economies in the colonies centered around whatever chief good they could supply to the colonizer. The merchants and the mine and landowners sold the goods to Europe and kept the surplus, allowing them to grow rich. They used this wealth to take more land. They also used their wealth to buy art, jewels, or manufactured goods from Europe. They built churches and palaces. The surplus was not used to reinvest in the local communities or to foster development of a local economy. This created extreme dependence on trade with Europe, and great vulnerability to any shifts in the market. Later, when a resource dried up, the town around it died and was abandoned, leaving what was left of its original inhabitants destitute.

The amount of wealth taken from the colonies was immense, and it changed the world economy. By the year 1560, over 100 tons of gold had been taken from the Americas. However, silver, which would become the true prize, soon outweighed gold on ships headed back to Europe. By the year 1600, an estimated 25,000 tons of silver had been transported to Spain. The Potosí mines became the most stunning source of wealth for the Spanish in all their empire. At their peak, around 1600, the Potosí mines produced more than all the silver mines operating in the world combined. John TePaske, in *A New World of Gold and Silver*, estimated that mines in Potosí and the surrounding area alone produced 22,695 metric tons of fine silver between 1545 and 1823. This is an even more astounding number when you consider that in the year 1500 all of Europe had only 37,500 tons of silver, and 3500 tons of gold.

American gold and especially silver transformed Europe and fed the development of the modern European market economy leading to increases in commerce and manufacturing. Ship after ship took wealth back to the colonizers. This gold and silver didn't stay there, however; it merely passed through. This was because the Spanish and Portuguese crowns were in a great amount of debt, in part because they continued to fight expensive religious wars. The gold and silver they received went to bankers throughout Europe as payment for debts.

Aside from debt, the flush of gold and silver also gave Spain and Portugal new purchasing power. They were not industrialized nations, so they increasingly began to buy manufactured goods like textiles or weapons from other places. Trade with China, India, and other European nations increased. The Industrial Revolution began in Europe because it was fed by American gold and silver. Gold and silver could be exchanged for manufactured goods. As the economy grew, the population of Europe did as well. The transformation of Europe was under way.

The transfer of stolen wealth from the Indigenous peoples in Latin America to Europe allowed capitalism to become the new economic system replacing feudalism. The European expansion that happened in the 18th century would not have been possible without the gold and silver stolen from the Americas. The modern world's economic system is built off the pillage of Latin America and the Caribbean, the genocide and forced labor of the Indigenous peoples, and as we will now see, the slave labor of Africans, all on stolen land.

AFRICANS IN LATIN AMERICA AND THE CARIBBEAN

The African slave trade added a new racial group to the Americas and Caribbean, weaving Africans into an already evolving demographic tapestry. This furthered the creation of complex new racial and cultural identities in the colonies. In some places, like Brazil, they and their descendants would become the majority population. Most people who receive a U.S. centric education are shocked to learn that the vast majority of Africans brought via the transatlantic slave trade were taken to Latin America and not to what would become the U.S.

Africans first arrived in the Americas and Caribbean during the conquest. They were enslaved workers brought by the *conquistadors* from Europe, or free men, descendants of the formerly enslaved in Europe, who came as explorers. When Native populations diminished due to disease and violence, the Europeans sought out an alternative source of labor. The African slave trade would meet that need.

The African slave trade provided the labor force that fueled the plantation economies in Brazil, Venezuela, and the Caribbean. In places like Peru, Ecuador, Argentina, and parts of Central America, African labor supplemented the *mita* system. African labor sadly became an essential fuel to both the Portuguese and Spanish colonial economies.

The transatlantic slave trade was the largest long-distance forced migration of people in recorded history, and likely the deadliest. The Atlantic slave trade, controlled by the Portuguese, took people from West and Central Africa to the Americas, beginning in the year 1526. The voyage across the Atlantic, known as the Middle Passage, was extremely perilous. Fifteen to twenty percent of those forced onto the ships died during the two-to-three-month-long crossing.

The people stolen from Africa were not a monolith. They spoke many different languages and came from different ethnic groups. It is estimated that around 12 million people over four centuries crossed the Atlantic. More than 10 million were taken to Latin America. About 4.8 million Africans went to just Brazil. To put this into another perspective, only 450,000 Africans were taken to what is now the U.S. Once in Latin America, the Africans endured cruel and dehumanizing conditions. Devastatingly, one-fifth to one-third died within three years of arrival.

The events of the time aligned in such a way that made Africans a desirable workforce in the colonies. The development of the slave trade in the colonies coincided with the opening of the West African coast for trade with the Portuguese. Commercial trade between Europe and West Africa increased and became more stable and dependable. The Africans had skills that were highly desired in the colonies. They were experienced at raising cattle, riding horses, iron and steel work, and mining. Aside from mining, these were things that the Native populations in the colonies had no prior knowledge of or experience in, creating a preference for African laborers. In places like Brazil, the native Tupi, who were semi-sedentary, were not accustomed to the systematic style of farm labor, making them an unreliable workforce. They often disappeared into the trees and escaped. Their knowledge of the landscape worked against the colonizers, something that could be alleviated by bringing in labor from a faraway place. Another especially important factor at the time was that due to centuries of contact between groups from Africa and the Iberian Peninsula, Africans had better immunity against the diseases that nearly wiped out the Natives.

Africans first went primarily to Spanish colonies in areas now known as Mexico and Peru and worked in a variety of industries. But, eventually, Brazil and the Caribbean came to rely on African slave labor most heavily. Most Africans who went to Brazil and the Caribbean worked on plantations. By the 1600s, the native population of Brazil was all but extinguished, and Africans replaced Indigenous peoples as the enslaved workforce.

The Portuguese required a steady stream of arrivals from Africa to maintain their plantations and agricultural exports. In the first 250 years of Brazil, about 70% of all new arrivals to the colony arrived enslaved. During the 17th century, almost as many slaves arrived in Brazil alone as arrived in Spanish America and the French and British sugar colonies combined. No other colonies imported as many enslaved Africans as Brazil. By 1810, more than 2.5 million slaves had entered Brazilian ports. Spanish America also utilized African slave labor, but to a different extent. Between the early 16th century and 1810, Spanish America received nearly one million Africans, or about 13% of all enslaved Africans brought into the Western Hemisphere by that point.

Africans enslaved in the colonies endured harsh conditions, especially on the plantations that dominated Brazil and the Caribbean. Plantation agriculture relied most strongly on slave labor, and the work on plantations was demanding. The enslaved labor force, which on Brazilian plantations could number from 60–100, were fed a poor diet and lived in small thatched or mud huts or barrack-like buildings. Slave owners chose to keep costs to a bare minimum, so clothing, shoes, and adequate food were scarce.

Slavery in the Spanish colonies was concentrated around mining and artisanal work until the late 18th century when

Cuban sugar and tobacco plantations grew, requiring increased slave labor. Because plantation labor grew later in the Spanish colonies, there was a higher percentage of African slaves in urban settings working as servants, manual laborers, vendors, and artisans. In large cities like Caracas, Buenos Aires, Havana, Lima, and Quito, enslaved Africans made up between 10 and 25% of the populations. In these urban areas, the work was less brutal than on plantations, resulting in higher life expectancies and increased birthrates for Africans and their descendants, although they no doubt endured abuse as well.

Despite the harsh oppression Africans and their descendants lived under, they formed families and maintained connections to their culture through music, dance, and spirituality. Africans resisted their captivity in clever ways, including purposefully sabotaging work, killing livestock, faking illness to slow production, and through more overt acts like rebellions and revolts. These revolts began during the Middle Passage. On at least 300 voyages the Africans attempted to overthrow the crew. During colonization, a small number were able to escape from slavery and formed free communities called *quilombos* in Brazil and *palenques* in Spanish America. These communities often formed alliances with local Indigenous groups, early showings of solidarity against oppression. By the 1670s, there were as many as 20,000 runaways in Brazil, with Palmares in Alagoas being the largest *quilombo*. Mexico, New Granada, Ecuador, and Venezuela all had large *palenques* that lasted several years.

In an economy designed to enrich the colonizer to the maximum benefit, African lives were viewed more as a commodity than as a life. To justify the oppression and treatment of Africans, the Europeans again leaned on their religion to provide an answer as to why it was acceptable to treat other human beings so callously. And just like in the case of the Indigenous populations, the church gave its blessing. The Catholic Church owned more slaves than any other group, business, or family in the Americas. By the 18th century the Society of Jesus was the single largest owner of slaves. Again, religion and colonialism intertwined to support the growth of capitalism, and European control and dominance. Again, the wealth garnered from murder and stolen labor, this time of Africans, became a fuel to building the capitalist economy of Europe and the world as we know it today.

THE LEGACY OF COLONIZATION

Colonialism in Latin America and the Caribbean lasted for three centuries. From the arrival of the Europeans in 1492 to the establishment of colonies by 1600 to independence in the early 1800s, there were three centuries of Spanish and Portuguese colonizers imposing their culture, language, religion, social structures, worldviews, and deep belief in their racial superiority onto Indigenous people and enslaved Africans. This was not only a colonization of the land, and people, but also of the body and the psyche, as these beliefs were implanted and reinforced over and over again.

The dominance of colonialism lasts long after the official period in history ends. Colonial structures and mindsets were embedded into the culture and ways of life, even in the way we came to view ourselves in racial and national terms. The structure of our modern world is built on colonialism, yet we rarely learn our true history, what colonialism has done to us, and what was taken.

Reflection and deconstruction

★ Were you ever taught about colonialism in Latin America? Was this information readily available to you or did you seek it out?

★ In the education you received, how were the colonizers portrayed? How were Indigenous peoples and Africans portrayed? How much emphasis was there on the experience of the Indigenous peoples or Africans?

★ How does increasing your knowledge of the true history of colonialism in Latin America impact how you view the world? Are there areas you want to learn more about?

★ Who benefits when we are not taught our history, our ancestors' accomplishments, and our contributions to the world system?

CHAPTER 3

CREATING RACE IN THE AMERICAS

Race is one of the lasting legacies of the colonial period in both Latin America and the U.S.

Despite how long the concept of race has been around it continues to be a confusing topic for many of us Latinxs. Race can very much feel like a moving target, and that is because it sort of is. Race is constructed differently in different places to meet the needs of those in power. Race is not a static well-defined concept. Its meanings can be shifted, changed, and renegotiated as needed to maintain systems of power and control, as has been done since its inception.

Race was invented. It is an imagined social and political concept where people are assigned a group based on observation of their physical features. Mainly skin color, but eye color, facial features, and hair texture are also considered.

These "racial groups" are given a social meaning by being placed into a hierarchy where the white group is at the top. The fewer physical features associated with whiteness you have, the further you move down the hierarchy into the margins of society, away from social, economic, and political power. When it comes to access to power and resources, and unfortunately even when it comes to your right to exist, it doesn't matter much how you conceptualize your own race, but how others perceive you.

During the colonial period, race was used to provide the

colonizers with another legitimizing narrative that could give cover for the atrocities they were committing. Initially they relied on religion. They described Natives and Africans as savage or beastly people who needed to be converted to Christianity to save their souls from eternal hell. As the colonies developed, and different groups mixed both sexually and culturally, the colonizers needed something more—especially because they were vastly outnumbered. Their answer to their problem was to impose a social structure that allowed a small group of wealthy European elites to maintain power and resources at the top of the social order and relegated the Indigenous peoples, Africans, and their descendants to the bottom.

Because race is viewed differently in the U.S. than it is in Latin American and Caribbean countries, racial identity can become a point of confusion.

To better understand how this came to be we will explore how concepts of race in Latin America were introduced and then shifted over time. First with the example of the Spanish racial caste hierarchy, and then by exploring the *mestizaje* and nationalism projects that took place in many Latin American countries. We will then contrast this to how race has been constructed in the U.S.

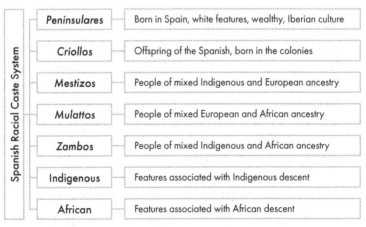

Spanish Racial Caste System		
	Peninsulares	Born in Spain, white features, wealthy, Iberian culture
	Criollos	Offspring of the Spanish, born in the colonies
	Mestizos	People of mixed Indigenous and European ancestry
	Mulattos	People of mixed European and African ancestry
	Zambos	People of mixed Indigenous and African ancestry
	Indigenous	Features associated with Indigenous descent
	African	Features associated with African descent

Figure 3.1: The construction of race in Latin America: The caste system

The racial caste system was born during the colonial era in Latin America, because the colonizers wanted to keep strict distinctions between white Europeans and everyone else. In the Spanish version of an ideal world, society would have had three separate categories: Spanish, Indigenous, and Africans, defined as rulers, tributaries, and slaves. However, as inevitable racial mixing occurred, new categories of social identity were formed. Each identity category was assigned a social value within the hierarchical system, and caste was officially recorded on the baptismal register.

By the early 1800s, mixed race people were more than half of the population, primarily mixed Indigenous and Spanish, or *mestizos* as they were referred to. Although the Spanish were in the minority, they maintained political, social, and economic power at the top of the hierarchy and the Indigenous people and Africans were kept at the bottom. This was supported by racial narratives that espoused their natural inferiority.

Placement in the hierarchy determined access to noble titles, legal class divisions, participation in government, and access to education. This hierarchy created incentive for people to distance themselves from Indigenous or African origins to have better access to resources and improved social status. For example, someone marked as Indigenous would benefit from becoming *mestizo* because it would relieve them of the burden of the *mita*. They could do this by petitioning the court, or the more likely option, by leaving their community.

There was a degree of fluidity to the castes, and as colonial society developed some people were allowed to move up in status to fill gaps. Some elite *mulattos* were even allowed to purchase whiteness from the Spanish crown in a process called *gracias al sacar*. Once they were officially seen as white, they were allowed to practice professions they had previously been forbidden from. Described in the book *Purchasing Whiteness* by Ann Twinam, decrees received from the Spanish crown stated their "defect from birth" was erased and they were granted the rights associated with whiteness. Practices such as *gracias al sacar* allowed the caste system to blend with the class system. Signs of wealth are associated with higher castes even if the person's phenotype alone would place them lower on the scale. This is something that continues today in Latin America, making whiteness more flexible than it is in the U.S.

Unlike the U.S., racial mixing was a generally accepted part of Spanish colonial society and understood to be a normal byproduct of these different groups living together in the colonies. The hierarchal categories were even depicted in paintings known as *Las Castas*. These paintings from the 18th century reflected colonial society and showed families from different castes in their home life. The paintings were often a four-by-four grid with each row depicting four different families of different racial mixtures. Families with a white European parent were often in the top row, with lower castes shown in bottom rows. Black women were often depicted as being aggressive towards their husbands in the paintings, while *mestiza* women were often depicted as submissive.

Las Castas reflected society and portrayed different racial identities as distinct from others. They influenced attitudes towards different races, increasing stigma towards those with African ancestry. They also showed that women who had children with white men or someone of a higher caste improved their caste and that of their children. In the Spanish colonies, mixed children could be accepted as legitimate heirs, inherit land or wealth, and improve their status. Children could receive racial benefits from their higher status parent. This type of racial advancement was not available to mixed-race children in the U.S., who were seen as illegitimate and assigned the social status of the parent with lesser status.[1]

---

1   U.S. president Thomas Jefferson produced multiple children with Sally Hemmings, whom he enslaved. Sally was only one-quarter Black, the daughter of Betty Hemmings, who was biracial, and white slave owner John Wayles. Sally's children, who were one-eighth Black, were not acknowledged as Jefferson's children, and they were also enslaved by him.

FROM CASTE TO NATIONAL
IDENTITY AND *MESTIZAJE*

As colonialism came to an end, this overt classification system lost its usefulness to those in power, which meant that concepts of race needed to change. The *criollos* wanted independence from Spain. Under colonization they were considered second-class citizens due to being born in the colonies and not Europe. *Criollos* were kept from the highest positions of power that were reserved for *peninsulares*. At this time, monarchies were also falling out of favor as a ruling system. The *criollos* wanted to fully participate in the developing capitalist system unrestricted by European monarchies. But although the *criollos* were big in power and resources, they were small in numbers. They needed a unifying rallying cry to bring non-whites to their cause. Like the revolutionaries in the British colonies who would form the U.S., the *criollos* were influenced by the ideas of the European Enlightenment. They began to promote the concept of forming independent nation-states.

The *criollos* promised that any man born in the Americas would be an equal citizen in the new nation-states, not just white Europeans. In 1813, famous Mexican Revolutionary leader, who was of Indigenous, Spanish, and African descent, José María Morelos y Pavon, proclaimed, "May slavery be banished forever together with the distinction between castes, all remaining equal, so Americans may only be distinguished by vice or virtue." The revolution promised an end to racial stratification, slavery, and peonage.[2] With independence came brand new national identities distinct from Europe: *Mexicano, Peruano, Nicaragüense, Brasileño*[3] and so on. Citizenship promised greater social and economic mobility regardless

---

2   This differed from the revolution that formed the U.S. which excluded non-whites from citizenship. It wasn't until the 14th amendment was ratified in 1868 that African Americans were defined as equal citizens under the law.

3   Most countries in Latin America abolished slavery by 1850. Cuba and Brazil were the last countries in Latin America to abolish slavery, finally ending the abhorrent institution in 1886 and 1888 respectively.

of race, but this did not materialize. Racist beliefs, practices, and social stratification persisted, just less openly. These new countries inherited colonial structures that had been built on domination and justified by an intense belief in the natural inferiority of large sections of the population. This wasn't something those at the top were willing to give up despite their promises to.

In the 20th century the ideology of *mestizaje* emerged. Like the caste system, *mestizaje* was designed to promote the goals of those in power. Simply put, those goals had now changed, and a new narrative was needed. *Mestizaje* is an ideological concept that tells a story about national identity based on three key points. First, the story celebrates a romanticized Indigenous past that seems to gently end at conquest. Second, the story tells of the creation of the *mestizo*, a symbol of the blending of two unique cultures, the Indigenous and the European, to form a unique new citizen. And third, the story reveals a modern nation with some Indigenous elements but with a Westernized culture and a Western future. *Mestizaje* as a project sought to unite a nation under a common, selectively edited, history and identity.

Mestizaje was promoted by Latin American elites to assist with nation building. The goal was to accomplish Western modernization of Latin American countries, modeled on European countries and the U.S. Intellectuals of the time believed that to be a truly developed nation, a homogeneous society was necessary. *Mestizaje* sought to strengthen national identity, while downplaying racial and ethnic differences, and class and political divides. *Mestizaje* embraced racial mixture in Latin American countries and affirmed that this history of mixture was a benefit to the nation and population.

Mexican philosopher and Minister of Education José Vasconcelos in *La Raza Cósmica* (*The Cosmic Race*) energized *mestizaje* ideology by proposing that the mix of races on earth would give rise to a superior fifth universal race or cosmic race where the inferior would be absorbed and improved on by the superior. This proposition required assimilating

Indigenous groups into a new modern Western society and diluting African heritage. *Mestizaje* is sometimes praised for its embrace of racial blending without much attention to its underlying racism.

Vasconcelos described Latin America as the ideal place for an emergence of the cosmic race due to Latin American spirituality, openness, and tolerance, which he contrasted to the English refusal to mix with other races. *Mestizaje* provided Mexican leaders with a way for the state to resist U.S. and European assertions of cultural and genetic superiority and assert their own potential. The idea of the future supremacy of a *mestizo* race grew popular, and the *mestizo*, the person of mixed race, became the prototypical citizen in Latin American countries.

Mestizaje was promoted to different degrees in each country. It received the most institutional support in Mexico, and Brazil, where it was called racial democracy. The governments promoted the narrative of *mestizaje* through education and the arts. In Mexico, *Indigenismo* policies were developed to better integrate the Indigenous groups into the new Mexican society through things like cultural education, and economic development programs. You can see the influence of these policies in public murals and architecture around Mexico today. State-funded murals by Diego Rivera, José Clemente Orozco, and David Alfaro Siqueiros combined European styles like cubism, symbolism, and expressionism with Indigenous techniques, colors, symbols, and popular figures especially from the Mexica (Aztec) and Maya.

Some countries like Argentina, Uruguay, Costa Rica, and to some degree Chile were less interested.[4] Countries in the

---

4   In 2021, during a meeting with Spanish Prime Minister, the President of Argentina Alberto Fernandez stated, *"Los Mexicanos salieron de los Indios, los Brasileros de la selva, pero los Argentinos de los barcos. Eran barcos que venian de Europa,"* which means "The Mexicans came from the Indians, the Brazilians came from the jungle, but we Argentines came from ships. And they were ships that came from Europe" which shows us the persistence of white supremacist attitudes, and denial of Indigenous and African people in Argentina.

Andean region like Peru, Ecuador, and Bolivia had weaker attempts to utilize *mestizaje* as a nation-building project, and in the case of Guatemala it only became a priority when it was used to try to quell the Indigenous rights movements by dismissing their need for specific cultural rights. In their promotion of *mestizaje* countries also promoted the goal to *mejorar la raza,* meaning to improve the race, by increasing the amount of white blood in the population. Countries like Mexico and Argentina actively sought out European immigration called *blanqueamiento.* The goal was to dilute the Indigenous and African blood. The saying *mejorar la raza* is still used today when people are encouraged to choose partners with lighter skin to produce lighter children.

While promotion of *mestizaje* appeared to be a method of embracing the racial diversity of Latin America, it perpetrated erasure and allowed for a cover-up of on-going racism. Although indigeneity is venerated in the marketing of *mestizaje*, Indigenous peoples were spoken of as something of the past or as an impediment to a better more Western future. Indigenous peoples are reduced to an ingredient in *mestizos* whose influence on dominant culture is recognized, but their continued existence, distinctiveness, and agency is ignored. The ideology of *mestizaje* in fact clashes with the continued existence of distinct Indigenous groups with their own unique and distinct cultures and ways of life.

There are approximately 50 million Indigenous people who belong to at least 500 different ethnic groups in Latin America today. Indigenous peoples continue to be abused by Latin American governments, discriminated against, displaced, disproportionately live in poverty, and face continued assault on their lands, and ways of life. *Mestizaje* attempted to force assimilation, but Indigenous peoples in Latin America have continued to utilize legal, political, and social processes to organize, mobilize, and fight for their rights.[5] Especially

---

5   For more on Indigenous movements see *Struggle for Indigenous Rights in Latin America* (2012), edited by Nancy Grey Postero and Leon Zamosc.

since the 1960s, Indigenous activism has been a force in Latin America.

Only Brazil and Cuba acknowledged the contribution of Africans to the country in their *mestizaje* projects. All others focused only on the European-Indigenous hybrid—a near total African erasure, and a shock considering how many people of African ancestry live in Latin America. African contributions to building Latin America are largely ignored, and Afro-Latinxs continue to be commonly excluded from Latinidad, even though The Project on Ethnicity and Race in Latin America estimates there are about 130 million Afro-descendants in Latin America. *Mestizaje* allows for the denial of anti-Black racism in Latin America, holding to the myth that a people of mixed race cannot be racist.[6]

Mestizaje became a way to absolve Latin America from its racism. It promoted the idea of unified countries, each made up of a unique homogeneous people of mixed descent who have overcome racism through unity and formed a superior race. Tanya Katerí Hernández uses the term "racially innocent" to describe Latin America's resistance to address the deep-rooted racial inequality that exists.

Refusal to see racism doesn't mean it doesn't exist. The denial of racism by Latinxs exists to such a degree that in Tanya Katerí Hernández's book, *Racial Innocence: Unmasking Latino Anti-Black Bias and the Struggle for Equality*, the opening line had to be "Latinos can be racist." Being a Latino doesn't absolve someone from racism. So, although many Latin American countries and people claim to have overcome issues of race to be free of racism, and see this as a uniquely American problem, we know that racist beliefs, practices, and policies persist.

---

6   For more on Africans in Latin America see *Beyond Slavery: The Multilayered Legacy of Africans in Latin America and the Caribbean* (2007), edited by Darién J. Davis, and *Black in Latin America* (2011), by Henry Louis Gates Jr.

COLORISM

Most Latinx people have experienced colorism, either directly or indirectly. Colorism comes alive in hospital delivery rooms when a *tía* delights at a newborn baby's green eyes or when someone looks behind the baby's ears to see what color they'll be. Colorism is rampant in societies where whiteness can change your life path for the better. Colorism is the preference for lighter skin tones even if that isn't always said out loud directly. Like Cherrie Moraga (1983) noted in her essay *La Guera*:

> I was "la guera": fair-skinned. Born with the features of my Chicana mother, but the skin of my Anglo father, I had it made. No one ever quite told me this (that light was right), but I knew that being light was something valued in my family.

Colorism leads to discrimination against those with darker skin tones and is a symptom of our community internalizing society's racism. A 2022 Pew Research Center study found that those with darker skin color experience greater Latinx on Latinx discrimination. Luis Noe-Bustamante writes, "about a quarter of Latino adults say they have personally experienced discrimination or unfair treatment from other Latinos. Having darker skin and being born outside the U.S. are associated with an increased chance of experiencing this type of discrimination."

In Latin American countries, Afro-Latinxs continue to experience higher rates of poverty, higher rates of health problems, lower literacy rates, and less educational attainment than those with lighter skin privilege. Because the history of oppression and slavery in Latin America is denied or minimized, these differences are explained away using old tropes of "laziness" or "incompetence" to justify the current circumstances of Afro-Latinxs.

For many Latinx people in the U.S., colorism comes right at us through our *abuela*'s TV. Anyone who questions racism in Latin American society and culture can easily check out one of Latin America's most successful cultural products and exports—the *telenovela*—to see colorism in action. As Sofía Aguilar writes:

> For most of my childhood and adolescence, if my abuela wasn't cooking me fideo or heating up a can of Juanita's pozole, she was watching Mexican telenovelas on T... they all looked identical to me—the overacted hysteria, the plot twists you always saw coming (how many times can a single person turn out not to be dead?), and always, the all-white cast of actors with darker-skinned people only in servitude or poverty, never with any agency of their own.

Another clue into the issue of colorism is to simply listen to the comments made in casual daily conversation. *Hay que mejorar la raza, casate con un güero*, we need to better the race, marry a blonde/white guy, or *vete por la sombra, te vas a poner prieta*, get in the shade, you're going to get dark (ugly). These comments, often made passively and without a second thought, signal a strongly rooted bias related to race that has been internalized by the culture over the centuries. While being called *mi negrita* by a loved one when you have a tan can be considered a term of endearment, it can't be separated from the history of racism that exists and underlies its teasing nature.

The caste systems that existed during colonization created societies structured around a hierarchy based on race and allowed white Europeans to maintain power in Latin America even after colonialism ended. *Mestizaje* later served as a nation-building project, but also to hide the continued privilege that white Europeans enjoyed. Indigenous peoples and Afro-Latinxs have been kept at the bottom of the social order, experiencing continued discrimination and exclusion.

Mestizaje accomplished many of its goals, including presenting an outward-facing homogeneous national and racial identity. However, it accomplished this by hiding the reality of the racial and cultural stratification present. A study by Edward Telles and Denia Garcia found that *mestizaje* ideology continues to be embraced in many Latin American countries and is viewed positively. *Mestizaje* is one reason why when Latinx people are asked about their race they are unsure of what to answer. Latin American countries generally excluded race on their own census forms. In the U.S., Latinx people are told they're an ethnicity but are also reminded that they definitely shouldn't see themselves as white. The white category on most forms says "White—not of Hispanic origin."

A 2021 Pew Research Center study found that when Latinos in the U.S. are asked their race the majority will answer with either a pan-ethnic label like Hispanic or Latino or claim their race as a nationality, naming the country of origin of their ancestors. In Latin America we shifted away from racialization, and in the U.S. we are excluded from the dominant racial identities, leaving us uncertain of where we belong when it comes to questions of race.

RACE IN THE U.S.

Unlike Latin American countries, the U.S. has always had a more purist relationship to race that revolves around exclusion. In the U.S., race historically has been a binary Black or white concept.[7] In fact, in the 1900s several laws in the U.S. went as far as to proclaim that anyone who had any African ancestry was Black, known as the one-drop rule. This meant that all it takes is one drop of African blood to make you Black or more importantly to keep you from the benefits of whiteness.

Different definitions of race mean someone immigrating from Cuba, Venezuela, the Dominican Republic, and so on can come to the U.S. and be racialized as Black by U.S. society,

---

7   The Black and white racial binary in the U.S. is currently being disrupted by the fast-growing Latinx population in the U.S. and confusion about how to count us on the Census compounded by our own confusion as to what boxes we should pick. These confusions are especially apparent for Afro-Latinxs, who most often fall through the cracks of our classification system. In 2019, there were 2.2 million Afro-Latinxs in the U.S., a 121% increase from 2000 to 2019. Afro-Latinxs grew at almost twice the rate of non-Black Latinos over the same period.

despite not being seen as Black in their home country, and never having perceived of themselves as a Black person. Race plays an important role in American society and daily living, yet it rests on how others perceive you, and cares little about how you identify yourself. Once in the U.S., a Black body will be treated as such, and ethnicity and culture come secondary, if they're even acknowledged at all.

While *mestizaje* drove the creation of national identity in several Latin American countries, Indigenous and African people have been excluded from the central nation-building narratives that patriotic Americans hold dear. American imaginations conjure up visions of manifest destiny, the god-given right to expand west across North America. Stories about taming the Wild West, lone cowboys,[8] and democracy and capitalism reaching from sea to shining sea define the American cultural consciousness. Rarely spoken of is the forced removal and ethnic cleansing of Native Americans from their lands. American children are taught that George Washington, this nation's first president, was an honorable man who never told a lie. Rarely are they taught that he was a prolific slaver or that as a general he ordered the first genocidal campaign in U.S. history. He commanded hundreds of troops to ensure the complete destruction of Iroquoia to clear lands for settler occupation.

In the U.S., the prototypical citizen, the white man, is always centered. When the U.S. was established, the white man was the only person who was considered a full citizen and even a full person. Enslaved people were counted as three-fifths of a person, and women were excluded from voting, owning land, and many other rights associated with full citizenship. This value is exemplified by the fact that every single president in the history of the U.S., except one, has been a white male. Reflective Democracy Campaign found in a 2021

---

8   Before there was the American cowboy, there was the *vaquero*. The original *vaqueros* were largely Indigenous American and Black men, first trained by the Spanish, who could wrangle cattle on horseback. The word lasso comes from the Spanish word for rope, *lazo*.

study that the U.S. is under white male minority rule. Despite being only 30% of the population, white men made up 56% of the U.S. House of Representatives and 68% of the Senate; 76% of governors and 90% of elected sheriffs were also white men.

To be a white man became synonymous with what it means to be a true and full American. A brown or Black-skinned Latinx person, even when "white-washed" or "coconut,"[9] one can never be fully accepted as white and will always be othered. A white Latinx person can potentially be accepted into the privileged class of whiteness, but it will ask of them the same thing it asked of the Italians and the Irish—to leave their cultural heritage behind.

The U.S. approach to race has historically been one of separation and exclusion. Integration of minority racial groups has only come about through the strategic activism of Black, Latinx, and other minority groups during the Civil Rights Movement. Decades of lobbying Congress, massive demonstrations like the 1963 March on Washington, pressure campaigns including the Montgomery Bus Boycott and the Delano Grape Strike and Boycott, and carefully selected high-profile lawsuits like Mendez v. Westminster and Brown v. the Board of Education led to the legal end of segregation and discrimination based on race, national origin, religion, and gender. In the U.S., whiteness has never given up power without a fight. Even when Latinx, Black, and brown people have been allowed to integrate into previously white-only spaces we quickly learn that integration isn't synonymous with acceptance. We are left to contend with the white supremacy culture we find there. This has drastic impacts on the social and emotional well-being of Latinx people of all types, as will be explored in the next chapter.

---

9   Some have described being called a coconut by white people meaning a person is "brown on the outside but white on the inside" and therefore "one of the good ones."

Reflection and deconstruction

★ As a Latinx person, how do you identify racially? How is your race perceived by others? Does it ever change?

★ How has your skin color impacted your experience as a Latinx person within your family? Community? Society?

★ What did you learn in your family regarding race and skin color? How has this influenced you?

★ How do you define what it means to be an American in the U.S.? Where do these beliefs come from?

★ What is your relationship to whiteness?

CHAPTER 4

MAKING THE INVISIBLE VISIBLE

Unlearning White Supremacy Culture and Seeing Systems of Oppression

You ask me what color my skin tone is, and I will tell you: It is a morning cafecito con leche with your abuelita. It is a carmelo tint that looks unreal, painted beautifully on my flesh. I do not burn with the sun; I evolve right before my very eyes. My Brown skin is beautiful. In the winter it becomes a lighter shade, the color of walnuts, and in the summer it darkens. I have to change my makeup with the seasons to match my beautiful, evolving skin tone, because my skin is supernatural.

—PRISCA DORCAS MOJICA RODRÍGUEZ, *FOR BROWN GIRLS WITH SHARP EDGES AND TENDER HEARTS: A LOVE LETTER TO WOMEN OF COLOR*

TO BEGIN...

Discussions about race, privilege, and oppression can be difficult. These topics tend to trigger discomfort, shame, rage, and other powerful emotions. Although we did not create the harmful systems we live in, we do have a responsibility to challenge them if we hope to reshape the world into one where all people can live free from institutional harm. Only when we deconstruct the influence they have had on us can we begin to take our power back. We must be critical of the world we live in. As we will see, accepting the status quo means accepting social conditions designed to keep us down.

While reading this you may notice yourself experiencing strong emotional reactions. These reactions can make us turn away from the material or want to reject it outright. This avoidance provides a short-term benefit by relieving us of distress, or from the work of having to look at a lot of aspects of life in a different way. But it hurts more in the long run. Over time, avoidance paralyzes us and decreases our capacity to engage in the necessary work of healing and creating avenues for social change. There is no easy way to do hard things.

WHITE SUPREMACY CULTURE

The dominant culture in the U.S. is white supremacy culture, but we just see it as what is normal. Whiteness is the American default identity, and the standard to which every other group is compared. As Toni Morrison so wisely expressed (Izadi 2019), "In this country, American means white. Everybody else has to hyphenate." A social psychology study on implicit bias, conducted by Thierry Devos and Mahzarin R. Banaji, found that non-white Americans are consistently associated less often with the label "American" than white Americans. The *researchers* concludes, "American is implicitly synonymous with being White."

This hidden reality can really do a number on our emotional well-being and sense of self, because most people just want to feel normal. We want to belong. Feeling as if we have similarities and things in common with others gives us a sense of connection, belonging, and safety. When what keeps us from fitting in with the status quo and ideas of "normalcy" is core to our culture and identity we can experience painful rejection because we get the sense that we are wrong in some way. Defective even.

If we do not expose white supremacy culture, we are at risk. As Judith H. Katz, Ed.D. stated when she called attention to the fact that white culture was the foundation of the counseling theories used to train mental health clinicians, "the need to make White culture explicit is significant when we realize that it exists but has rarely been acknowledged or investigated." When counselors or helpers try to make people adjust to society's values without recognizing that they are enforcing assimilation, they perpetuate cultural oppression, and harm Latinx people.

White culture includes the ideas, values, norms, habits, rules, assumptions, and beliefs held by the descendants of White Europeans in the U.S. People who identify as white are rarely made to think about their racial identity because they live within a culture where whiteness has been normalized. Some people even joke about the lack of culture whites have, proving just how invisible it is. There is nothing wrong with White Europeans having their own worldview and culture, but it becomes a problem when it is expressed as superior to all others, as is done in the U.S.

White supremacy culture, the idea that white culture is superior, is a product of racism that exists at a societal level. It functions from the belief system that people in the white racial group are superior and therefore deserve the privilege. People who are in the other racial groups are seen as less than. Their lack of power and resources is explained to be the result of their supposed natural inferiority. Forcing colonized populations to accept white supremacy culture perpetuates the colonization of the mind.

The logic of white supremacy culture is one of the long-lasting mental edifices of colonialism that is made real in our lives by the way it influences laws, policies, and institutions. It influences the way we relate to each other, and even the way we see ourselves and people like us. Although white supremacy is an idea, we live in the world it created every day.

White supremacy culture seeps into our brains and bodies, whether we benefit from it or not. If we were fish in the ocean, white supremacy culture would be the water. We have no choice but to swim in it and take it in. It's in how we are socialized. There is no way to avoid absorbing some of the belief systems, values, distortions, or biases of this culture during our lives. It becomes a wish to have a smaller European nose, disdain for other Latinx people who we think behave too stereotypically and make us look bad. It's in devaluing Latinx art, movies, or music. They are labeled as not as good as what is produced by whites and Europeans. It becomes a negative attitude by Latinx people in the U.S. towards immigrants, scapegoating them as a drain on our resources, forgetting they are *nuestra gente*, our people.

If we are not made aware of white supremacy culture, we may begin to overly identify with the dominant culture and accept the supposed inferiority of our own. White supremacy culture is cleverly hidden, and not often spoken about. This is what gives it so much power. When something creates our daily reality in such a powerful way, and can stay almost invisible, it is harder to deconstruct and to challenge. Instead of saying, "this is white culture" we say, "this is normal." It is "normal" to pack a peanut butter and jelly sandwich for school, and not a burrito filled with last night's leftovers. It is "normal" for your mom to speak perfect English, and not have an accent. It is normal to have straight blonde hair, and never need to sit for hours in a salon having your dark hair straightened. It is normal to live in a home with both parents and one sibling exactly, and it is not normal to share a home with your grandparents, cousins, and other relatives.

Internalized white supremacy culture becomes anti-Black attitudes, and the denial of Afro-Latinxs and Latinegrxs. It becomes embarrassment at Indigenous traditions, remedies, or ways of life. It becomes refusal to speak Indigenous languages or Spanish to our children. White supremacy culture will have Latinx people buying into stereotypes about other oppressed people. Worst of all, it means we do all of this, often without even knowing we're upholding white supremacy culture. It is only when we are made aware of the water that we can start to see it, to question it, to challenge it, to change it, to be liberated from it. As Black writer James Baldwin wrote, "It took many years of vomiting up all the filth I'd been taught about myself, and half-believed, before I was able to walk on the earth as though I had a right to be here."

CALLING OUT THE QUALITIES OF WHITE SUPREMACY CULTURE IN THE U.S.

Internalizing parts of white supremacy culture does harm our physical, emotional, and spiritual health, and this must be resolved to be healthy and well. Most of the rest of this chapter explores the qualities, beliefs, and values of dominant white culture expressed by Tema Okun, a diversity trainer and educator, as well as other information from mental health texts regarding cross-cultural counseling. I have also included common ways these values impact us Latinxs with knowledge gained from my clinical practice with Latinxs and folks from other marginalized identities, my work with students and supervisees, and my own lived experience. Consider that these values are not the natural way of the world, or the "right" way for a society to operate, they are just a set of cultural values we've come to see as normal. We can reject them to whatever degree we choose, especially if they are in opposition to our Latinx culture or make us feel bad about ourselves and our people. Use the reflection and deconstruction questions to go deeper, and consider how internalizing these has impacted you and people like you.

Perfectionism

The belief that perfection is attainable, and perfection should be the goal. We are taught that attaining perfection gives us value and worth as a person. Making mistakes, not being perfect, or not doing things perfectly is assumed to reflect poor character. It is the belief that there is one right or perfect way to do things.

Internalizing perfectionism can look like...
An inner voice that becomes a harsh critic that berates us for mistakes, and our lack of perfection. Thoughts of "I have to be perfect," "I cannot make mistakes," "If I make a mistake, I am a failure," "If I make a mistake, I am a bad person." Holding ourselves and others to unrealistic standards. Devaluing, minimizing, or not recognizing our efforts towards a goal because only perfect completion matters. Not valuing our mistakes, and what we learn from just trying things out. Feelings of unworthiness. Never feeling good enough, no matter how hard we try. Deep despair at our lack of perfection.

Reflection and deconstruction

★ How has perfectionism impacted you?

★ Whose standards are you trying to meet when you strive for perfection? Did you decide on these standards or were they externally imposed?

★ How can you reject beliefs related to perfectionism within yourself, and in your work towards liberation for your community?

★ Can you shift to allowing yourself to be good enough in different areas of your life? What does good enough mean to you?

Dominance and superiority

The belief that dominance equals superiority and value. The belief that one superior group can rightfully maintain power in society over other groups, because those groups are "less advanced" or "less civilized." The superior group can define normal, control institutions, and impose their standards on others. The unquestioned belief that those who hold power are in that position because they must know best, are the most qualified, and are the smartest. The unquestioned belief that those in positions of power make decisions in everyone's best interest. This dominance and superiority also extend to power over natural resources and animals for the benefit of the dominant group. Nature is viewed as something to be conquered, controlled, or monetized to the benefit of those with power, and not as something that human beings are a part of.

Internalizing dominance and superiority can look like...
Defending, upholding, and supporting the power structure when it actively harms marginalized groups. Assuming leaders and those in power know best and shouldn't be questioned. Preference for the dominant group even when you are not a member of it. Trying to change yourself to be more like those in power with the hope that you will attain some of that power or gain acceptance or validation from those in power. Allowing others to make decisions on your behalf. The belief that "they must know better than me" or "what I know about this doesn't count" or "why bother, there's nothing I can do about it." Giving your power away to others, or not recognizing it to begin with.

Reflection and deconstruction

★ Are there other ways to be powerful aside from force and domination over others? What are alternative ways of seeing power?

★ In what ways do you minimize or ignore the power you have?

★ What would it look like for you to step fully into your personal power? What about collective power?

★ How do dominance and superiority mindsets impact the human relationship with the natural world?

★ What is your connection to earth and nature?

Objectivity

The belief that there is such a thing as being completely objective or neutral. Denial that this faux objectivity or neutrality upholds the current power structures and allows harm to continue. A preference for rationality, and emotional control. Displays of emotions are seen as bad, and a sign of loss of control and lack of ability to think logically. Emotions are not seen as valid or helpful. A preference for logic.

Internalizing objectivity can look like...

Ignoring how someone's environments, life experiences, and personal characteristics influence how they perceive the world. Devaluing emotional intelligence and rejecting or ignoring our emotions. Judgment of others who display emotions. Ignoring how emotions provide important information to us about our environment. A disconnect from our internal world, and creativity. Devaluing creativity in favor of systematic and rational practices. Using neutrality to avoid engaging in social issues. Staying neutral in situations of injustice, because we do not feel personally impacted, or because we fear that taking a stance against the current power structure will bring us harm. Belief that knowledge produced scientifically is the only knowledge of value, and the stories, traditions, or ways passed down by our culture are not as valuable or as good.

Reflection and deconstruction

★ Brazilian philosopher Paulo Freire said, "Washing one's hands of the conflict between the powerful and the powerless means to side with the powerful, not to be neutral." What does this mean to you? Have you been neutral in the face of others' oppression?

★ Have you ever used reason and logic to shut down or push away your emotions?

★ Have you ever been told your feelings are wrong because they aren't logical? If so, why? Who does this serve and who does it harm?

★ How can you learn to value your emotional intelligence, creativity, and the wisdom of your body and culture just as much as other more accepted forms of knowledge?

Binary thinking

A pattern of thinking where things are seen as having two absolute categories. Even complex ideas or problems are reduced to binaries. This can also be called black/white and all-or-nothing thinking. This type of rigid thinking leads to difficulty seeing nuance, grey areas, and accepting that multiple things can be true at once and can feed depression, anxiety, and other difficulties.

Internalizing either/or thinking can look like...
Thoughts can include:

· "I am either a good person or a bad person, and there is no in-between."
· "If I do something wrong or make a mistake, I am a bad person or a failure."
· "If I acknowledge something wrong or harmful that someone has done, I am saying they are a 100% bad person."
· "There is only right or wrong, and things have to be one or the other."
· "You're either with me or against me."

Binary thinking can lead to discomfort with conflict, or difficulty finding resolution for problems due to decreased flexibility, less willingness to understand others' perspectives, or inability to make compromise. There may be difficulty accepting that others can experience something differently from you, and that their truth is also valid. All-or-nothing thinking can lead us to treating ourselves and others harshly. We may have difficulty with cognitive flexibility, and reduced empathy. Either/or thinking can lead to isolation because we have difficulty being in relationship with people who do not share our values or beliefs, leading us to reject them entirely. We think "you're either with me or against me," making it difficult to form community due to the vast diversity that exists within all people.

Reflection and deconstruction

★ How does either/or thinking, all-or-nothing thinking, or black and white thinking show up in your life?

★ Instead of an "either/or thinking style," can you incorporate a "both/and" style of thinking?

★ Both/and thinking is when we can acknowledge that multiple things can be true at once, and we can feel more than one emotion about something at a time, creating space for acceptance of differences. Examples can include...

☆ "I love *tacos de lengua* (beef tongue tacos), and my sister hates them. Both of our opinions are valid and okay."

☆ "Jose has been supportive to me in my life, and has done things that have hurt me. Both can be true, and acknowledging harm doesn't negate the help or support they've shown me. It also doesn't mean I have to pretend that those harms didn't happen."

☆ "I can be sad that I went through something hard, and proud that I survived. I can hold two different, even opposing, emotions at once."

☆ "I can love my parents and have boundaries with them."

☆ "I can be there for my family, and say no sometimes."

★ Based on the examples above, can you create a sentence using both/and thinking that applies to an area of your life?

★ What is it like for you to hold two truths at once?

★ Are there certain situations or certain people where you find this especially difficult? Why? What does that tell you?

Capitalism and quantity over quality

The belief that our goal should always be to do more, achieve more, accomplish more, produce more, earn more, own more, or consume more. The emphasis on quantity, production, and ownership supersedes everything else, including the quality of our work, quality of our relationships, our personal needs, and the needs of others.

Gordon Gekko sums up many of these values perfectly when he professes the following in the 1987 movie *Wall Street*:

> In my book, you either do it right or you get eliminated... The point is, ladies and gentleman, that greed, for lack of a better word, is good. Greed is right, greed works. Greed clarifies, cuts through, and captures the essence of the evolutionary spirit. Greed, in all of its forms; greed for life, for money, for love, knowledge has marked the upward surge of mankind. And greed, you mark my words, will not only save Teldar Paper, but that other malfunctioning corporation called the USA.

Capitalism infuses daily life with a great sense of urgency, and pressure to achieve things quickly while being ruled by deadlines. Success is always in doing more, and there is a preference for quantitatively measurable goals within specific timeframes. Only things that can be measured or make money have value. Anything and everything can be commodified. Resources are more likely to be directed towards things that have a measurable impact and generate a profit. If the benefit of something is difficult to measure such as with art education, community gardens, or after-school programming, it is less likely to get continuous funding.

Internalizing capitalism and quantity
over quality can look like...

- "The more I produce the more valuable I am as a person."
- "I get my value from external achievement."
- "I must always be active, or productive, or I am worthless."
- "I am only as valuable as my credentials, titles, or positions."
- "Time is money."

Difficulty resting, slowing down, or engaging in pleasurable activities that are not deemed to be productive. Devaluing relationships. Devaluing processes such as spending time with others, resolving conflicts, discussions, learning groups, mutual support, or forms of labor that are not tied to wages or earning more money. Belief that rest should be earned, and that busyness demonstrates personal value. Personal self-worth is tied to obtaining material possessions. A continuous focus on growth, change, and the future and difficulty being present and accepting or valuing where you are now. Strong physical discomfort when sitting or relaxing.

Reflection and deconstruction

★ What is your relationship to rest and stillness?

★ What happens when you try to rest?

★ What examples of rest did you have or not have? Why?

★ How much of your self-esteem or personal value comes from production, achievement, consumption, or busyness?

Individualism

Individualism is as American as apple pie or pulling yourself up by your bootstraps. Heavily influenced by the Protestant Work Ethic,[1] American individualism values personal responsibility, personal freedoms, independence, and autonomy. This belief system encourages people to be seen as individuals, not as members of social groups. People are supposed to be judged based on their individual merit. Personal success is because of merit, meaning those who are seen as successful are often assumed to be good, moral, or deserving. This provides a useful cover for privilege, and the unearned advantages that some enjoy. Successful people are assumed to be worthy of the rewards the system provides them.

Individualism also means that everyone, in theory, takes full responsibility for any negative outcomes in their lives.[2] This is weaponized against people from marginalized backgrounds who can then be blamed for lack of success, and feeds into beliefs regarding inferiority and deficit in Latinx communities. Complex social issues like poverty, homelessness, or

---

1   The Protestant Work Ethic teaches that hard work brings success. Good fortune is seen as a sign of God's favor. This idea links wealth with morality and poverty with immorality.

2   During the Great Recession in 2008, the U.S. government gave banks $500 billion in taxpayer-funded bailout money, because they were deemed too big to fail, while six million households lost their homes to foreclosure. Families were expected to take personal responsibility for taking on bad mortgages, but banks were saved despite being responsible for selling defective financial products like subprime mortgages. According to UnidosUS, "the housing crisis at the center of the Great Recession stripped a collective 66% of wealth from the Latino community."

addiction are often reduced to personal failures.[3] This belief system ignores the natural interdependence of humanity and importance of history and social forces. By only considering the individual, and not considering their interconnections such as family, environment, or social group membership, we ignore how privileged identities advantage some while marginalization disadvantages others. There is an emphasis on the individual's interests over group or community interests. There is a strong focus on individual rights, and a disregard for social responsibility, community, or environmental responsibility. The focus on individualism leads to a harsh denial of the existence of racism, sexism, ableism, or other oppressive social systems, and a defensiveness when these issues are brought up.

Internalizing individualism can look like...

- "Every man for himself."
- "I have to win, so others have to lose."
- "You always have to look out for yourself first."
- "I can't depend on anyone."
- "Asking for help is a sign of failure, or not being good enough."
- "People who ask for help are needy and incompetent."
- "I had it hard so you should too."

Devaluing interdependence, and seeing the Latinx focus on community as codependent, unhealthy, or toxic. Placing great emphasis on the self, and ignoring the interconnection

---

3   In the U.S., when substance use was perceived to be an "inner city" (code for Black, brown, or other socially undesirable group) problem it was met with the War on Drugs policies beginning in 1970. This created harsh legal penalties with mandatory minimum sentences, and funding to create a militarized police force. Substance users and sellers were criminals. Later, when the opiate crisis impacted white Americans at higher rates, it was treated as a public health crisis. Opiate users were seen as victims of the pharmaceutical industry.

between self, environment, family, community, culture, history, ancestors, and spirituality. Focusing on competition over cooperation. Difficulty celebrating others' accomplishments due to seeing their success as your personal loss, or an affront to your own place in the imagined competition of life. Not wanting to help others, and feeling as if everyone should be on their own. Seeing help and assistance as something other people must earn and be worthy of.

Reflection and deconstruction

★ How have you internalized the toxic messages of extreme individualism?

★ How do you feel when you ask for help? How do you feel when you help others?

★ Do you see your growth and healing journey as an individual pursuit? Why or why not?

★ Can our healing be separated from community and culture? Why or why not?

★ Consider a time you succeeded or accomplished something important to you. Who else contributed to your success? Could you have done this without others?

Right to comfort (for those with power)

Those in power have a strong belief in their right to emotional comfort, leading to avoidance of open conflict and the ability to engage in discussions related to social issues, oppression, and privilege. The person or group causing discomfort or conflict is often blamed, seen as violating social norms related to behavior, politeness, or professionalism. Those calling attention to issues such as racism or sexism may experience blame, retaliation, isolation, or exclusion.

Internalizing the right to comfort (for those with power) can look like...

- "I can't speak up, because it means I'm confronting someone, and behaving aggressively."
- "If something makes me or others uncomfortable it's automatically bad."
- "If a conversation makes me feel bad, they must be saying I am a bad person."
- "I shouldn't have to talk about, think about, or learn about something if it makes me feel uncomfortable."
- "Get over it."

Avoidance of conversations about race, religion, politics, or other "taboo" topics. Taking others' emotions or responses to situations personally. Expectation that people who have been harmed by oppression and state violence only advocate for themselves or resist in appropriate, nice, or socially acceptable ways. Discounting the violence endured by Latinx people through colonialism, racism, sexism, economic oppression, anti-immigrant policies, while expecting the continued compliance with the norms and expectations of these systems. Telling people who have been harmed to not be angry.

Reflection and deconstruction

★ How do you feel when you speak up about social issues? What emotions come up? How does your body feel?

★ How can you lean into discomfort or create a tolerance for it so that you can do your highest healing work?

★ Are you willing to create discomfort in service of your own and others' liberation? Can you do this in community with others?

Aesthetics

Music and art based on European culture is valued, held up as a model, and wins awards. Women's beauty standards are based on Eurocentric features such as being blonde, blue-eyed, thin, and young. Men's attractiveness is based on athletic ability, appearing powerful, or being successful economically.

Internalizing this aesthetic

Acceptance of society's dominant beauty standards can show up as body dysmorphia, an internal sense of shame or disgust about one's appearance, and even self-harm. We may go to extreme lengths to embody Eurocentric beauty standards such as over-spending on beauty products, skin-bleaching cream, and even plastic surgery. We may reject as partners those who do not meet a Eurocentric ideal without questioning first what we actually like versus what we are taught to like. We may try to buy our way into whiteness by wearing name brands we associate with being white or having a higher social status.

Reflection and deconstruction

★ How have you been influenced by Eurocentric aesthetic standards?

★ What is your relationship to art, music, and other cultural products created by non-white people?

★ Has this changed or evolved over time?

White supremacy culture is complex, and unraveling it piece by piece allows us to begin deconstructing how it has influenced us, and allows us to decide if we want to continue holding these value systems and beliefs. We can unlearn what has been forced on us, and make space to relearn values and beliefs that are nourishing to our spirt, well-being, and health.

SYSTEMS OF OPPRESSION

Racism isn't the only system of oppression we deal with in the U.S. There are plenty of white people who experience oppression, and there are plenty of Latinx people who have privilege. Racism is one system of oppression, and it works in tandem with others. Black feminist writer bell hooks, in *Feminist Theory: From Margin to Center*, encouraged us to see how different systems like race, gender, and class interlock and support each other. She boldly named our society "a political system of imperialist, white supremacist, capitalist patriarchy," giving us a tool to understand the complexity of our reality.

It's important to understand how systems function. Michelle Johnson, a licensed clinical social worker, of Dismantling Racism organization, explained in a workshop I was fortunate enough to attend how oppression operates. She said that in all systems of oppression the policies, practices, and protocols of social institutions advantage, serve, resource, and validate the powerful social group. Those who are excluded from this social group are excluded, disadvantaged, and exploited. The dominant social group is advantaged by this system politically, socially, and economically. The dominant social group has greater power and control within this system, and this power shapes the dominant culture. In the system of racism, inclusion or exclusion is based on race, the dominant group is white people, and they get to impose their standards onto others. Society is structured to their benefit at the expense of everyone else. The less powerful social groups are Black, Indigenous and Native, Latinx, Asian, and anyone else who isn't seen as white.

Other systems of oppression include sexism, ableism, ageism, heterosexism, classism, and capitalism. Each system advantages one powerful social group over several others. For every oppressed group, there is a privileged group that benefits from their oppression. For every privileged group, there are several oppressed groups being held down by the system. All oppressed people suffer from limitations, not personal limitations, but limitations imposed by the system that prevent them from fully developing their abilities and capacities and from being able to truly express their thoughts, feelings, and needs.

Think...who would my grandfather have been if he had been able to finish school and hadn't had to leave to start working to support his family? Who would my grandmother have been if she had had the chance to do something other than be a wife and mother? What would she have chosen? Who could my dad have been if he hadn't been undocumented, and could have worked a secure job? Who could my sister have been if she had lived in a safe neighborhood? Who would I be if I had had all the resources, support, and encouragement?

Everyone deserves to be nurtured and supported. To have the opportunity to fulfill their capacities. This is one element of justice. And justice can heal and transform.

Mapping your place in the systems of oppression

System of oppression	Benefitting	Disadvantaging
Racism	White folks	Black, Indigenous, and other people of color
Patriarchy	Cisgender men	Women, trans people, non-binary people, gender non-conforming people
Heterosexism	Heterosexual folks	Lesbian, gay, bisexual, asexual, polyamorous, aromantic folks
Ageism	Adults	Babies, children, adolescents, teens, older adults/elderly
Classism	Wealthy, owners of capital	Poor, working class
Ableism	Able-bodied	Physical disability, mental health disability, cognitive disability, chronic illness or pain, temporarily disabled, pregnant

cont.

System of oppression	Benefitting	Disadvantaging
Christian supremacy	Christians	Jews, Muslims, Hindus, Buddhists, Indigenous spiritualists, and those who practice animism, shamanism, polytheism
American imperialism	Natural born U.S. citizen, native English speaker	Undocumented person, Deferred Action for Childhood Arrivals (DACA) recipient, immigrant, refugee, naturalized citizen, non-English speaker, English as a second language

Because everyone is a member of multiple social groups at once, each representing a different aspect of identity (e.g. race, sex, gender, sexuality, citizenship status, economic class, age), we can experience both privilege and oppression simultaneously. This is succinctly put by Afro-Peruvian writer Kayla Popuchet Quesada when she says, "All Latinos are nationally oppressed, but not all Latinos are racially or ethnically oppressed."

Although all Latinx people experience oppression to some degree, they also oppress each other, and create within-group discrimination. The more marginalized groups a person is a member of, the more severe their oppression becomes and the further into society's margins they go, leaving them without protection, resources, and recognition of their humanity. Two people can each be Latinx and have completely different lived experiences due to difference in gender, class, race, or more.

Reflection and deconstruction

★ What are your social identities?

☆ Race

☆ Ethnicity

- ☆ Socioeconomic status
- ☆ Gender
- ☆ Sex
- ☆ Sexual orientation
- ☆ National origin
- ☆ First language
- ☆ Disability
- ☆ Age
- ☆ Religion/spirituality

★ Which of these identities most influence your daily living?

★ Which of these identities do you think about the most often? The least often?

★ Which of these identities have the strongest influence on how you perceive yourself? What about how others perceive you?

★ Which of these identities create disadvantages? Which of these identities bring you closer to power or privilege?

CHAPTER 5

SOUL WOUNDS

Colonization was more than a historical event. It was a collective trauma. Our Indigenous and African ancestors' natural life courses were disrupted, and they were forced into a new reality. Surviving the historical traumas of genocide, slavery, forced assimilation, displacement, and discrimination created lasting wounds on Latinx people. These wounds have radiated psychic and spiritual pain across generations. Fortitude through challenge led to unique survival strategies that over time became cultural strengths and intergenerational resilience. How do we begin to talk about the impact something of this scale had on us as a people? How do we start to talk about our pain so that we can begin to heal from it?

The mental health field, led by the American Psychiatric Association (APA), offers one way of describing our pain: as a mental health disorder. The *Diagnostic and Statistical Manual of Mental Disorders (DSM)* names all mental health disorders currently recognized by the APA, along with a list of symptoms and diagnosing criteria. In defining disorders this way the APA uses a medical model for diagnoses. This choice by the APA follows a long history of the psychology field in the U.S. vying to be seen as a legitimate hard science akin to biology and physics.

Classifying mental health struggles as disorders suits a medical model, and dominant American culture's desire to make everything quantifiable, by making mental health appear to be clear cut and easily definable. It also creates mental health stigma. It sends a message that having a mental health disorder means something is inherently wrong with you, that you might be broken or defective in some way. This leads many to shy away from engaging with the mental health field for fear of being labeled as mentally ill.

The *DSM* relies heavily on a mental health condition's impact on a person's functioning. Functioning mainly rests on someone's ability to participate in their community as a worker, or student, and maintain a level of independence in their daily living. When psychological distress is severe enough to disrupt these functions, they are considered diagnosable.

Disorders are identified because they are seen as a deviation from what is considered "normal." Normal in the U.S., as we have already discussed, is synonymous with white cultural behavior, thinking, and expectations. Again, whiteness is the thing we are measured against. If we understand our pain and distress through this white Western lens, we will use terms such as "major depressive disorder" or "generalized anxiety disorder." We will accept the idea that "something is wrong with me." While the list of symptoms for these disorders may accurately describe some of what we are feeling, it provides no context or explanation as to why we might be feeling this way. It's kind of like being told you have heart disease, and when you ask "why?" the response is "because your chest hurts."

Having a mental health diagnosis can have many benefits. A diagnosis can be validating for some. It can also be required to qualify for some mental health services, or to get accommodation at work or school. However, these terms are not appropriate to describe the deep collective wounding that has happened under colonization and the accumulation of trauma since.

For us Latinxs, our liberation includes stating the why, and not allowing this part of our experience to be silenced or hidden any longer. Current mental health disorders don't account for our experience as a community, and they ignore the historical context under which harm occurred. They don't capture the insidious effects of life under the weight of continued domination, racism, and discrimination. These terms are at best too narrow to capture what Latinx people experience, and at worst intentionally hide the real reasons for our suffering. Latinxs must understand that the typical American mental health system that has historically seen our culture as an impediment to emotional well-being rather than an asset to it may not be able to meet our needs for healing.

By taking control of our own healing and liberation, we can reject the framework that measures health and wellness against white supremacist normalcy. What is abnormal, and what is in fact deeply unnatural, is colonialism and all that it brought on us. The question then becomes, "Is there a normal way to respond to collective historical traumas?" It is not those who are harmed who are deviating from the natural or civilized, but the current organization of power in the world that breaks with humanity.

We are not disordered—capitalism, racism, patriarchy, heteronormativity, xenophobia, and the interlocking systems of oppression are the disorders. We are not sick, and we are not mentally ill. We are individuals, families, communities, and people living with the impact of a deep unnatural wounding. Despite these atrocities, we have survived and pushed forward together, even when wounded and in pain. Even in our deepest suffering, Latinx people find a collective humanity, resilience, strength, and even humor. We deny the oppressor of their deepest desire—to make us less than human.

NAMING THE HISTORICAL TRAUMA

Healing the wounds of colonization requires us to first acknowledge the context where the wounding occurred. We can look to Indigenous scholars who are leaders and knowledge creators in the fields of healing and liberation to start this process. Lakota social worker and mental health expert Maria Yellow Horse Brave Heart introduced the term "historical trauma" to explain the wounds of Indigenous peoples of the Americas, defined as the original inhabitants of the land area now known as the U.S., Canada, Mexico, Central, and South America, and their descendants.

According to Dr. Brave Heart, historical trauma is the cumulative emotional and psychological wounding across generations, including the lifespan, which emanates from massive group trauma. Historical trauma is made even worse by the on-going racism, discrimination, and oppression that the groups who first experienced the trauma and their descendants continue to face. Naming what we have experienced as historical trauma provides the necessary context to explain our experience.

The historical trauma of colonization, the forceful takeover and exploitation of the Americas, Caribbean, and much of the African continent by European nations and later the U.S., laid the groundwork for an environment where Indigenous peoples, Africans, and their descendants were highly vulnerable to further trauma, displacement, and experience continued discrimination.

COLLECTIVE TRAUMAS EXPERIENCED BY LATINXS IN THE U.S.

An example of postcolonial collective trauma is what followed after 1848 when the U.S. won the Mexican-American war. The Treaty of Guadalupe Hidalgo gave the U.S. 55% of Mexican territory. This included the present-day states of California, Nevada, Utah, New Mexico, Texas, most of Arizona and Colorado, and parts of Oklahoma, Kansas, and Wyoming. Mexicans living in these territories were placed under the control of a new colonial master.[1] Many lost rights to their land despite land rights being guaranteed in the treaty.

Soon after the war, immigration to the U.S. by Mexicans

---

1   The Latinx population continues to be concentrated in these areas in the southwest, although the 2020 census does show population spread into areas that haven't historically had large Latinx population areas. North and South Dakota have the fastest rates of growth in their Latinx populations since 2010.

became popular. Mexicans were recruited by companies like the Southern Pacific Railroad to be exploited as cheap labor. Increased immigration led to the growth of anti-Mexican and Latinx sentiments. Latinxs in the U.S. were banned from white establishments and lived in segregated poor urban barrios. Even when they held U.S. citizenship, Latinx people were treated as unwelcome foreigners. Stereotypes grew, describing Latinxs as lazy, stupid, and irrational. These perceived flaws were blamed on the Mexican culture creating a toxic narrative around Latinx people that continues today.

Latinx people living in the U.S. experience continued discrimination, and it makes us a target for violence. We have been a convenient scapegoat for the U.S.' problems for many generations. We have been blamed for increases in crime, disease, and economic problems. Our immigration to the U.S. has largely been treated like an infestation. Even in places where our roots run deeper than the existence of the United States of America we are treated as unwelcome. Because we are perceived as a threat, we are often met with violence. This has led to more experiences of collective trauma where we are targeted just for being Latinx. The negative impacts of this violence flow out through the community as we share the fear of being targeted. Trying to protect us, our parents tell us to keep our heads down, work hard, and not attract too much attention.

Other collective traumas

- Lynchings: During the late 19th and early 20th century, in the aftermath of the Mexican-American war, Latinx people were often the targets of mob-led terrorism. Lynchings occurred for "crimes" such as insulting white people or fraternizing with white women. In 1877, over 40 people were hanged for the murder of one white man in Texas. Most of the lynchings took place in Texas, California, Arizona, and New Mexico. Lynchings and mob violence are known to be one violent method used by white people to assert their control over the American west.

- Segregation: Beginning in the 1870s, Latinx students were forced to attend separate "Mexican schools" based on factors like skin color and last name. These schools were under-resourced and provided a substandard education. Parents in the southwest challenged segregation in court at the state level, but the practice wasn't ended until the U.S. Supreme Court decision in 1954 in Brown v. Board of Education that ended segregation in schools.

- Eugenic sterilization: In 1907, the nation's first Eugenic Sterilization law was passed. These laws were eventually passed in 32 states. This allowed the state to forcibly sterilize those deemed "unfit." In California, sterilization was disproportionately done to Latinx patients due to racist bias and sexist stereotypes, including labeling Latinas as "hyper-fertile," and to prevent "anchor babies." Puerto Rico had some of the highest rate of sterilization. By the 1960s, one-third of *puertorriqueñas* had been sterilized. Recently, in 2020, immigrants being detained in a privately operated detention center in Georgia filed a complaint due to a government-contracted doctor repeatedly performing sterilization procedures on women in Immigration and Customs Enforcement (ICE) custody without their knowledge or consent.

- Repatriation drives: In the 1930s, during the Great Depression, Latinx people became a scapegoat for the dire economic situation. The public thought Mexicans used too many resources and took jobs from white Americans, resulting in anti-Mexican hysteria. Mexicans were banned from certain jobs, and 1.8 million people were deported to Mexico. Around 60% of these people were American citizens born in the U.S. to immigrant parents. People were often rounded up in informal illegal raids on public places and were not given any due process. They were simply loaded onto buses or trains and sent to Mexico.

- U.S. Immigration and Customs Enforcement (ICE) and Border Patrol: From the 1900s into the 1960s, white immigrants who entered the country illegally faced virtually no threat of deportation. They could legally work and were eligible for public benefits. Today, Latinx people face far harsher consequences for unauthorized entry. ICE is tasked with the location, detention, and deportation of undocumented immigrants. Latinx people have been targeted by this increasingly militarized and heavily funded federal agency. In 2017, ICE had a budget of $3.8 billion. Latinx people are the targets of aggressive raids and excessive immigration enforcement. In 2013, 96.7% of all deportations were of Latinx descent. Nearly one quarter of all Latinxs personally know someone who was deported or detained by immigration authorities. Since the 1990s, the U.S.–Mexico border has been militarized into a war zone.

- Gun violence: Two of the most horrific mass shootings to occur in the U.S. happened in Latinx communities. In 2019, a domestic terrorist targeted Latinxs in a mass shooting in El Paso, Texas, killing 23 people and injuring 22 others. The shooter posted a manifesto stating he was targeting "the Hispanic Invasion of Texas." The El Paso shooting is the deadliest attack on Latinx people in modern American history. In Uvalde, Texas, where the community is 82% Latinx, 19 children and two teachers were killed at Robb Elementary School. Law enforcement arrived within three minutes of the gunman entering the school but failed to enter the school for over one hour and 14 minutes. This was a clear violation of established police procedures initiated after Columbine which direct law enforcement to immediately engage a school shooter. Latinx communities are disproportionately at risk for gun violence. From 1999 to 2020, an estimated 74,522 Latinx people in the U.S. died from gun violence.

Reflection and deconstruction

★ Have you experienced the ripple effect of any of these other collective traumas?

★ Are there other collective traumatic events that you, your family, or community have been impacted by? How?

ENFERMEDADES DEL ALMA/THE SOUL WOUNDS

As Latino/a/xs we are very familiar with *enfermedades del alma* (illnesses of the soul). We know that outside forces can harm our spirit. This is why some of us try to protect our babies from *mal de ojo* or other spiritual attacks. Spiritual harm can create imbalance that manifests as illnesses of the mind or body. Some of us seek out *curanderxs* or healers to treat illnesses like *susto* or *espante*. We use *limpias*, medicinal plants, herbal teas or baths, and prayer to help us recover when our soul has been harmed. This is because we know that sometimes our illness has a spiritual component beyond what Western medicine can treat. And so, it makes sense that the violence of colonization could also harm the spirit in ways we haven't recognized.

North American Indigenous scholars have named this type of *enfermedad del alma* the soul wound. Native American psychologists Eduardo Duran and Bonnie Duran, in *Native American Postcolonial Psychology*, described the soul wound as the unhealed trauma that travels from one generation to the next. Duran and Duran state that the trauma is cumulative and becomes more severe with each generation when it goes unacknowledged and unhealed. The soul wound is an ancestral hurt that harms the spirit and must be treated holistically, incorporating mind, body, spirit, and culture.

Both historical trauma and soul wounding give us the necessary language to approach the healing that is needed for our Latinx community. Scholars such as Dr. Maria Yellow Horse Brave Heart, Teresa Evans-Campbell, and Les B. Whitbeck have conceptualized how historical trauma presents in the descendants of Indigenous people, while Antonio L. Estrada has explored how historical trauma can present in Mexican-Americans specifically. Dr. Joy DeGruy, in her book *Post Traumatic Slave Syndrome*, described responses to historical trauma present in the descendants of those who were enslaved.

Because of the diversity within the Latinx community these wounds may appear differently in different communities or in different people, but the following list represents common reactions to historical trauma and signs of soul wounding as theorized by scholars of historical trauma.

Fractured sense of identity
Distorted self-image
Identity crises
Deep longing
Fatalism
Anger
Rage
Rejection of family or group culture
Lateral violence
Self-hatred
Internalized inferiority
Desire to assimilate
Sense of powerlessness
Lack of belonging
Domestic violence
Child abuse
Depression
Anxiety
Substance abuse
Shame
Unresolved grief
Spiritual imbalance
Desire to be like the oppressor
Racial mistrust
Racism
Transphobia
Sexism
Loss of collective identity
Susto

When we live with unhealed historical trauma we are split apart into pieces, with a fragmented identity, uncertain of how to be made whole. Uncertain if we can ever be whole, feel worthy, content, or at peace. We are hateful to ourselves, and others like us. Our inner voice is cruel and can be unrelenting. When we suffer with this soul wound, we cannot nurture the interconnectedness our family needs from us to be a healthy balanced supportive unit, and we struggle to find the balance in our own life that will support emotional and spiritual health. When we suffer from unhealed soul wounds, we pass the baton of trauma on to the next generation.

We must commit to facing these wounds and nurturing ourselves whole again. In her book, *Light in the Dark/Luz en lo Oscuro*, Chicana writer Gloria Anzaldúa calls this process the Coyolxauhqui imperative, named for the dismembered Mexica Goddess. Anzaldúa describes Coyolxauhqui imperative as follows:

> A struggle to reconstruct oneself and heal the sustos resulting from woundings, traumas, racism, and other acts of violation *que hechan pedazos nuestras almas*, split us, scatter our energies, and haunt us. The Coyolxauhqui imperative is the act of calling back those pieces of the self/soul that have been dispersed or lost, the act of mourning the losses that haunt us.

Colonialism separates. We may have found ourselves fragmented with splits between body, mind, spirit, and soul. In healing, we labor to call back the pieces of ourselves that have been lost or separated. We are called to see ourselves and to see our experiences from a different vantage point. We are called to reclaim what has gone missing. We must re-write our stories, our histories, to learn and unlearn, as we reconstruct ourselves towards wholeness. We must engage in the creative process of making something new out of the pieces.

Reflection and deconstruction

★ What are your beliefs regarding mental health?

★ How do you nurture balance and emotional wellness in your life?

★ Do you feel a connection to the concept of historical trauma?

★ If so, in what ways have you seen historical trauma and resulting soul wounding impact you, your family, your community, or others?

★ What are your different parts of self?

★ Think of identities (race, age, nationality, ability, languages, etc.), life roles (brother, sister, daughter, occupation, etc.), passions or interests (writer, painter, dreamer, disruptor, healer, etc.)? Also consider your child self, teen self, adult self, and the selves you could become in the future. How do these parts fit together?

★ Are there any parts of yourself that you reject? Why?

★ What is something new you can make from these parts? How can you relate to these parts of yourself in a new or different way? In a loving way?

★ What tools does your culture offer to help you cope with historical trauma, soul wounds, or emotional pain?

CHAPTER 6

LA CULTURA CURA

Grieving What Was Lost and Reclaiming What Remains

GRIEVING WHAT WAS LOST: LAND AND IDENTITY

The soul wounds of historical trauma give us a name and framework for understanding. We are now faced with the journey of healing. Healing is not really an endpoint or a final destination. Healing is a practice, with peaks and valleys that bring us closer to the fullness of life and into loving connection with all living things, including with ourselves. Healing means to be able to hold many truths at once, including the joy and vitality of life along with the darker realities of the world.

Along the healing journey we are often accompanied by grief as we come to realize what's been lost. Grief must be attended to. Everyone grieves differently, but some common ways grief can present itself are sadness, anxiety, guilt, anger, helplessness, longing, and physical pain. Grief fills the space left empty by who or what was lost. A byproduct of conscientization is that it can bring latent grief closer to the surface of our awareness, initiating mourning.

One major loss for Latinx people is land. Not in the sense of having lost a parcel of land or a piece of property (although this can of course be a part of it), but in the sense of feeling deeply rooted in the place you live, having a history, culture, and identity tied to the land you're on. Displacement from communities whose collective identity was intertwined with a territory began soon after conquest, and some of us have been in motion ever since. Forced migration complicates the natural grief process that comes after loss. Grieving can feel like letting go, which we often don't want to do when leaving was forced. This makes the loss difficult to resolve, and thus more likely to be passed on. Some of us are born into grief.

We Latinxs also grieve identity. Although many Latinx people have some Indigenous ancestry, over time many of us have become *mestizx* and lost kinship ties to communities and places. This process is referred to as de-tribalization or sometimes de-Indianization, because we have lost a core component of what it means to be Indigenous.

To live today as an Indigenous person means more than having a blood connection. It also means to be claimed by a people and belong to a place as a descendant of its original inhabitants. Indigeneity comes from the interconnections between a group of people, a territory, and a history. Many Latinxs on their journey of healing from historical trauma confront the loss of Indigenous identity and feel grief.

The loss of indigeneity can leave us overwhelmed and searching for answers. We grieve the loss of culture, history, community, place, language, and ways of life. We grieve things we cannot name. We feel a deep longing for ancestral connections. For Latinxs in the U.S. who struggle to find belonging within a racist American society, this can be especially painful, as we already struggle with the push and pull of assimilation. This pain and the accompanying distress leads some to think that claiming an Indigenous identity is a solution to the problem of belonging—not only for belonging, but also as a way of reasserting oneself from a place of pride, dignity, and resilience in the face of oppression and discrimination. Locating one's identity outside colonial frameworks, much like when the Chicano movement in the 1960s or the Taíno revival movement of the 1970s reclaimed indigeneity, can feel empowering.

However, a word of caution when it comes to reclaiming indigeneity. Indigeneity is not a simple racial or biological category. It is a collective social and political lived experience.

Indigenous nations have agency, autonomy, and the explicit right to determine their own futures and their own memberships. These rights are explicated in the United Nations Declaration on the Rights of Indigenous Peoples. Indigenous nations define their membership how they see fit. The idea that blood ties equate to an Indigenous identity comes from a concept known as blood quantum. Blood quantum was another tool used by the U.S. government to exert economic and cultural control over Indigenous peoples.

Blood quantum was imposed in 1884 by the U.S. Bureau of Indian Affairs. Blood quantum refers to the amount of so-called "Indian blood" that an individual possesses. The Bureau enforced a requirement that a person has to have at least 25% Indian blood quantum to be a tribal member. Blood quantum was created to decide lineage, and to limit the number of Natives eligible to receive benefits over time. Congress hoped to reduce the number of people who could make claims to land based on indigeneity.

The idea that blood ties equate to group membership fits in with the way identity has been constructed in the U.S. Remember the U.S. utilized the one-drop rule to decide if someone was Black, so the idea that a certain amount of blood relation equates to being a tribal member becomes an easy idea to follow when you're educated in the U.S. However, despite our acceptance of it, blood quantum is not an Indigenous nor a scientific idea, and not all Native nations use this idea in conceptualizing what it means to be an Indigenous person. As Megan Minoka Hill, Oneida Nation Wisconsin, has stated, "Defining citizenship is probably the most sovereign act a native nation can make."

To be an Indigenous person today is to be a part of a distinct group with collective ancestral ties to the land and natural resources where they live or from which they've been displaced. Identity, culture, livelihood, physical and spiritual well-being are inextricably linked to the land and its resources. To be an Indigenous person is also to live the politicized and marginalized experience of an Indigenous person who faces institutions and transnational capitalist systems designed to extinguish not only you, but your culture and ways of living.

The U.S. government has long engaged in policy and practices designed to end what they have called "The Indian Problem" using extermination, displacement, and forced assimilation.[1] Transnational corporations have often targeted Indigenous groups who interfere in their money-making environmentally destructive projects.[2] This specific form of oppression is something many Latinx people have the privilege of avoiding exactly because they are not seen as Indigenous or are no longer a member of these especially vulnerable groups.

As Latinx people not connected with a distinct Indigenous group, nation, tribe, *pueblo-*, to assert ourselves and claim an Indigenous identity over the voices of the Indigenous people would be to replicate the domination of colonization. Liberation will not happen if we do not do the work of unlearning the colonial mindset; we will fall into traps such as this one over and over. The colonized mind says, "I belong!" and claims ownership. The decolonized mind asks, "To whom do I belong?" And, "How can we work together?" Stepping back from the black and white colonial way of thinking opens us up to greater possibilities. We can honor multiple truths, such as recognizing that we have Indigenous ancestry *and* that our lived experiences are different from those of today's Indigenous peoples. Both of our existences are signs of resistance and persistence. Both matter, but they are not the same.

---

1 For a complete history of this see *An Indigenous Peoples' History of the United States* by Roxanne Dunbar-Ortiz.

2 Berta Cáceres, activist from the Lenca people in Honduras, and co-founder of the Council of Popular and Indigenous Organizations of Honduras, is a prime example of how Indigenous people are targeted by governments and corporations. In 2015, she waged a successful grassroots campaign against the construction of the Agua Zarca Dam. In 2016, after years of threats, she was assassinated in her home by U.S. trained special elite forces at the direction of the former president of the hydroelectric corporation, DESA, the former leader of the dam project.

Liberation comes from solidarity between different groups who respect and recognize differences where they exist, and commonalities where they exist. We can honor our Indigenous roots, talk to our ancestors, and rejoice in all the ways indigeneity has influenced Latin American cultures without minimizing our privilege, and the lived experiences of Indigenous peoples today.

MAKING SPACE TO MOURN

Allowing yourself to grieve your losses makes it more likely your later choices won't be motivated by an impulsive desire to escape from pain. Grief requires us to name our losses, and to engage in mourning. We light candles, build altars, plant flowers, pray, and sing to our grief. We write letters to our grief. We talk with others about our grief. Each of these acts of mourning takes us through the grief process.

Grief is not something we can measure, and despite popular ideas about grief, it doesn't have stages. Grief can be unpredictable, and change day to day or moment to moment. A model I use with my clients that we have found to be helpful comes from psychologist J. William Worden who explains that grief has four tasks. They are not to be done in any order, and grievers often go back and forth between them over time. Each task involves a range of emotions, and processes that are unique to each individual. Although this model was developed in regard to loss of a loved one the framework can be applied to other types of losses.

- Task one: To accept the reality of the loss.
  Name the losses.
- Task two: To process the pain of grief.
  Cry, write, pray, sing, talk, engage in rituals or ceremonies, connect with other grievers.
- Task three: To adjust to a world without who (or what) was lost.
  Adjustments can include deciding to learn new things

or skills, adapting to a change in how we perceive our-selves and our identity, updating our belief systems or spiritual practices.

- Task four: To find an enduring connection with who (or what) was lost while also embarking on a new life. Over time we find a balance between honoring our loss and moving forward into a full meaningful life lived in accordance with our values. We may find that the way we view the world, and our place in it, has changed and that this new perspective incorporates a lasting connection to who and what was lost.

Grieving will help us to locate our own historical memory without erasing or stepping over today's Indigenous peoples. When we push to escape from grief, we delay our healing. Grief requires mourning. When we mourn, we accept and allow for the grief to flow. On the other side, we find that we can learn to incorporate Indigenous wisdom without repli-cating oppression.

Reflection and deconstruction

★ What losses have you experienced due to historical trauma?

★ How can you practice mourning these losses?

★ What type of lasting or meaningful connection would you like to have to what was lost?

FINDING STRENGTH IN CULTURE

Mental health research has shown time and time again that our mental health and well-being are improved when we have a strong connection to our culture and ethnic identity.

Greater ethnic pride results in higher self-esteem and overall general well-being, while reducing anxiety, distress, depression, hopelessness, and substance abuse. Research also shows that a strong cultural identity is a protective factor against the negative impacts of racism and discrimination. Our culture and a positive view of ourselves and the people we belong to give us tools to cope with the challenges of existing as a minority in the U.S.

Culture is a healing medicine for the soul wounds. Embracing a worldview anchored in our Latinx cultural strengths provides us with a path to separating from the colonization of the mind. We must find our way back to a more Indigenous-informed worldview—a framework that teaches us to understand ourselves away from the gaze of the oppressor, to see ourselves in sacred relationship with the land, and with others. If we can embrace the gifts of our culture and reject assimilation, we can experience transformational healing.

What we may not often consider is that despite no longer being connected to our Indigenous or African communities through known kinship ties we still carry ancestral gifts in our cultural consciousness. Mesoamerican, Andean, and African culture is alive today, not only within communities that have maintained their Indigenous ways, but everywhere. We may be accustomed to calling these aspects of culture "traditional", but these are gifts from our past. Interwoven into our modern culture are Indigenous and African resources.

When we talk about reconnecting to an Indigenous worldview, we are not creating something completely new or taking what isn't ours, we are recognizing and building from what is already there. This is a process Dr. Manuel Zamarripa from the Institute of Chicana/o/x Psychology calls Re-indigenizing. Re-indigenizing helps us create a dream for the future that supports us and our community being healthy, well, and spiritually nourished, based on our Latinx culture while honoring our Indigenous and African roots.

Reflection and deconstruction

★ What makes you proud to be Latino, Latina, or Latinx?

★ What cultural gifts have you received from your family or community? How do these help you during times of adversity? How can culture support your healing?

TRANSCULTURATION

Today's Latinx culture carries many Indigenous and African influences. This is because during colonization, a process called transculturation occurred throughout Latin America and the Caribbean. Transculturation is a term created by Cuban anthropologist Fernando Ortiz in his analysis on the development of Cuban society and culture. Transculturation describes the merging over time of different cultures until they create something unified and new.

Try as they might, the Europeans were unable to eradicate and replace Indigenous and African culture, especially outside cities where European influence was the weakest. Instead, over the centuries, people lived side by side and each culture influenced the other. We hear this transculturation when we listen to *timba*, *samba*, *salsa*, *merengue*, *cumbia*, and other popular music originating in Latin America and the Caribbean. European guitar, African *conga* and *tambora* drums, native *gaita* flutes, and *maracas* were combined to create a wide range of new musical styles.

Transculturation shaped what many Latinxs hold as sacred. In Latin America and the Caribbean, a blending of Indigenous, African, and European religion and spirituality led to today's practices. Missionaries learned to accept Indigenous and African cultural influences in church festivities, seeing them as a way of attracting more people to Christianity. We continue to see this during Indigenous-rooted celebrations of today like *Dia de Los Muertos* in Mexico, *el Día de los Difuntos* in Ecuador,

La Feria de Barriletes Gigantes in Guatemala, and La Calabiuza in El Salvador, which all happen around the Catholic holiday All Saints Day.

Transculturation became a survival mechanism for many Indigenous and African practices. With Catholicism being forcibly imposed on the Indigenous and enslaved Africans, they often disguised their own traditions and beliefs behind Catholic saints and celebrations to avoid punishment. For example, when La Virgen de Guadalupe appeared she was believed to be Tonantzin, the Aztec Earth Goddess. The Spanish accepted her, dressed her as a Catholic figure, and built a church to her on top of a sacred site that was already a destination for pilgrimage for the Indigenous population. This allowed an Indigenous practice of pilgrimage to continue, but under the guise of a Catholic Virgin Mary. La Virgen later became the patron saint of Mexico and a symbol of protection for the Indigenous population, bringing even more Indigenous peoples and their practices into Catholicism. Symbols such as the addition of blood on Catholic crucifixion figures, a remnant of the Mexican belief of blood as life giving, or towns having their own patron saint, a remnant of Mesoamerican belief in local deities, are signs of these integrations.

Similar processes occurred in places like Cuba, the Dominican Republic, and Brazil where we see a blending of Catholicism with African spiritual traditions and culture. Religion was a sustaining force for the enslaved African populations. Santería, widely practiced today, is based on the rituals of the Yoruba and was developed by enslaved communities in Cuba. Gods and goddesses, called Orishas, each have a Catholic saint counterpart. For example, Obbatala, the deity responsible for human creation, is portrayed as both Saint Mercedes and Jesus Christ. This allowed Santería practitioners to pray openly to their own gods under the disguise of their Catholic counterpart. Music, dance, and spiritual embodiment play a large part in the Yoruban traditions that influenced Santería as well, and you can even hear the names of Orishas in many popular songs like Chango Ta' Veni by Machito or Para Oshun y

Yemaya by Hector Lavoe. Certain rhythms and specific dance movements correspond to different *Orishas*. Similar religious traditions formed in Brazil known as *Candomblé* and *Umbanda*. Despite these having millions of followers, most people continue to identify as Catholic due to the history of persecution of these religious practices.

Indigenous and African cultures have been an ever-present influence despite their continued devaluation. This mixture of cultures has shaped our psychology, giving us a worldview and traditions separate from the dominant Western ideals of individualism, competition, and dominance. Understanding ourselves from this perspective supports greater emotional well-being. When we consider common cultural features of Indigenous populations, we can easily see the overlap and influence these values have had on Latinx culture. There is great diversity among Indigenous groups of the Americas and Caribbean, but there are some common values, and many have a corresponding Latinx cultural value.

INDIGENOUS CULTURAL INFLUENCES ON LATINX CULTURE
Indigenous cultural value: Collectivism
The tribe, group, or family take precedence over the individual. Harmonious relationships and social networks have great importance and are vital to survival. Interdependence, cooperation, and participation are highly valued and obligatory. Honor and respect are gained by sharing, giving, and service to others.

Latinx cultural value: *Familismo, humildad, y responsibilidad*
Familismo or familism teaches us to place a strong emphasis on the family unit, including extended family such as godparents, close friends, or our community. The family's collective welfare is of primary importance, and individual needs are secondary. We are taught to feel a strong sense of obligation to our families, and to the collective well-being of all. Individuals

may sacrifice their own needs or wants to support the family. Loyalty, reciprocity, solidarity, and fulfillment of family obligations are at the core of *familismo*.

Humildad or humility is of high importance for many Latinx people. We are taught to not focus on our successes, but to instead recognize our shortcomings. *Humildad* teaches us not to be motivated by personal achievement or gain, but to instead find our motivation in upholding Latinx community values and being supportive to others. We are taught that selfishness is undesirable.

Responsibilidad or responsibility is taught to us from an early age. We are taught to be accountable for our actions, to be honest, and to keep our word. We are taught that our duty is to care for others, and that this is innate to us as Latinxs and comes from within.

In their most positive expression, *familismo*, *humildad*, and *responsibilidad* offer us meaning, fulfillment, and purpose. When our families are functioning well, we feel healthier, more secure, and have a rootedness that safely grounds us as we move towards fulfillment of our goals. Positive support from a network of people is one of the most valuable resources the Latinx community offers. These values also offer us resilience in the face of challenges, and tools to use in the face of discrimination.

Reflection and deconstruction

★ Every family has stories that teach us our family history, family legacy, and ways we have overcome hardships. What family stories do you know where these cultural values were evident? How did they help your family to overcome or to succeed?

★ How did your family teach these values? How can you honor these values in your own life?

★ Have you ever used connection to other Latinxs to help you navigate a difficult or challenging circumstance?

Indigenous cultural value: Focus on harmony and balance

Balance and harmony are seen as key to maintaining health and wellness in Indigenous cultures. On a personal level, this means balance and harmony between different aspects of self: the spiritual, emotional, mental, and physical. On a collective level, there is a focus on maintaining balance and harmony between the family members, within the community, and between the community and the greater collective. Imbalance and disharmony are seen as sources of illness. Caring for the different parts of self, and acts of support and love towards others maintain balance and harmony.

Latinx cultural value: *Personalismo y simpatia*

Personalismo describes our interactional style. As Latinxs we value people and relationships. We take great care to have respectful, warm interactions with others, even if it is just how we engage with someone else while in line at the grocery store. We avoid confrontation and conflict when possible, preferring to maintain a sense of harmony in relationships. We build rapport and connection with others and take the time to make even small interactions feel meaningful. We bring a sense of familiarity to interactions, which promotes trust and connection with others.

Simpatia describes our friendly nature. We are taught to be warm, gracious, and hospitable, and to openly express positive emotions over negative ones. We see these values in the way we treat visitors in our home, always offering *café, pan dulce*, sweet bread, and *plática*, conversation. We live this value through frequent get togethers with family and friends. We celebrate! We're festive! We emphasize our blessings, even in times of difficulty. We look for opportunities to laugh and smile together, and often use humor to make others feel at ease.

In their most positive expression, *simpatia* and *personalismo* help us to have meaningful relationships and positive experiences with others. These values, when they are honored, create a foundation for stable and healthy relationships, allowing for increased trust and intimacy with others. These values also offer us a way to have frequent positive social interactions, which have been shown to reduce stress, loneliness, and sadness, and increase hopefulness and joy.

Reflection and deconstruction

★ Think of those in your family or community to whom you feel a warm connection. How were these connections built? What did they do, or did you do, to make this so? How do you feel when you are around them?

★ What is your interactional style? How do you incorporate these values into your daily living or interactions?

Indigenous cultural value: Cosmovision[3]

Cosmovision refers to the conception that Indigenous peoples have, both collectively and individually, that the nature of reality is that everything is sacred and interconnected. Human beings exist in sacred unity and relationship with the natural world and a cosmic order. Life is controlled by unseen powers that are all encompassing, including gods and ancestors.

Latinx cultural values: Spirituality and *querencia*

Spirituality is highly valued in our culture and carries many messages from Indigenous cosmovision. Even when Latinxs do not consider themselves religious, we often keep a sense of connection and even devotion to something beyond us. Some Latinx people are religious, predominantly Catholic, but many

---

3   For a modern-day application of Indigenous cosmovision check out *Universal Declaration of the Rights of Mother Earth* from the World People's Conference on Climate Change and the Rights of Mother Earth, Cochabamba, Bolivia, 2010.

also have a connection with other spiritual realities, such as elements from nature, ancestors, spirits, or saints. Many Latinx people find the spiritual world to hold meaning, shape identity, and be the key to living our destiny and full purpose. We live this value when we pray, light candles, build altars, tend to our land and plants, spend time in nature, consult our elders, or ask our ancestors for guidance or protection. We live this value when we dream of or envision a better future for ourselves and our loved ones. When we engage in rituals, they signify our connection to the cosmic order, and our place among all of nature and creation. We open ourselves to both influence and be influenced by forces greater than us. Our spirituality teaches us that life is sacred, and we are on a spiritual journey towards wholeness.

Spirituality can be an anchor point to a strong cultural identity due to how deeply intertwined it is with our culture. Spiritual practices are a resource for coping with the stressors of life and give us a sense of higher purpose. Spirituality provides a sense of transcendent connectedness. It is well established in mental health research that spirituality increases optimism, resilience, and psychological well-being.

Querencia describes our history of deep connection to place. *Querencia*, described by Juan Estevan Arellano in his writings about his home in New Mexico, is the link between land and the culture of those who live on it. The land provides an anchor to the identity of the people, and the people are in communion with the land. A deep sense of inner well-being comes from knowing and understanding the land, and being a steward of the land that will one day be cared for by your children. Although many Latinx people have been historically displaced and forced to migrate, we create *querencia* wherever we land. We may not have vast landscapes when we've been pushed into urban settings, but we have our grandmother's backyard, the trees our grandfather watered, our mother's apartment. We build families and identity around places.

Reflection and deconstruction

★ What do you hold sacred?

★ What makes you feel connected to earth, nature, spirit, ancestors, or your god(s)?

★ What rituals, prayer, or ceremony do you practice that give your life meaning?

★ What gives you strength?

★ What is your sacred purpose?

★ Have you felt *querencia*? Have you or your family created a beloved place?

THE POLLUTION OF CULTURE

Sometimes in the exploration of culture we may find it difficult to access the positive aspects of our cultural healing resources because they have been muddied by difficult, harmful, or abusive relationships with our own families. Because our families are usually our entry point into our cultural heritage, we may want to reject those who've harmed us and our culture entirely. It can feel insincere to talk about *familismo* when our own family has let us down. Today's world and the systems we live within such as patriarchy and capitalism make it difficult for us to always live our cultural values in their most positive expressions. Here are some examples:

- *Familismo* + patriarchy: Men have higher status in family systems giving them authority, and power over women and children. This power corrupts and women are then expected to care for and sacrifice for men and the family without receiving the same in return, so there is imbalance in systems of reciprocity.
- *Familismo* + *simpatia* + patriarchy + capitalism: Violence

or abuse against women and children is excused, normalized, or ignored to "keep the peace." Because families may rely on men for economic survival there is fear of disrupting the family and losing economic support. According to a 2022 U.S. Government Accountability Office report, Latinas are the lowest paid workers in the U.S., making $.58 for every dollar white men earn, less than women from other ethnic or racial groups. This makes them especially economically vulnerable. Families are also sometimes encouraged to stay together even when abuse is present, due to beliefs about the importance of family. Family members are pressured to maintain peace within the family by not speaking up about abuse or harm. This results in a false peace. It may appear that the family is cohesive and strong, but it is at the expense of the physical, emotional, spiritual, and financial well-being of some.

- *Familismo* + racism: Latinx families experience discrimination and racism within the legal and immigration systems. Despite harm, we may choose to protect family members from racist systems, including potential deportation or police violence, by not seeking legal justice when family members engage in harm. This often means that victims feel a lack of protection or justice. Internally, racism can influence how family members who are Black or have stronger Indigenous features are treated.

THE NEED FOR ACCOUNTABILITY

Harm within the family system is a real and present issue and danger for some Latinxs, and this cannot be hidden or ignored. When we allow for toxic patterns or abuse to continue, we allow the intergenerational transmission of trauma and soul wounding to grow more severe and continue. To heal our soul wounds, our community, and to shape a society free from oppression, the Latinx culture must become a culture of accountability and transformational healing. When we call for accountability for harm done, and healing for victims, and are simultaneously challenging the conditions which have allowed abuse to exist in the first place, this change ripples forward. Change can end cycles of violence.

Accountability culture can begin by teaching our children to be accountable and responsible for their actions and choices, and to understand how they impact others. We can model this by being accountable ourselves. When we have harmed our children, even unintentionally, we can apologize to them for the harm caused, take accountability, seek repair, and show them that we can change our behavior. This is an act of liberatory healing. This is one of the greatest gifts we can give our children. We can teach them how to have safe, loving, respectful relationships free from abuse by giving them a safe and loving relationship free from abuse.

We can also create accountability culture by shifting from hierarchical relationships to a building collective where power is shared, each member is equally valued, and everyone's contributions are respected. We can respect each other's boundaries and commit to engaging and communicating in ways that are respectful.

We must also hold those who harm accountable. We cannot excuse or minimize abuse within our families. So often, victims of familial abuse are silenced and ignored or maybe worse, shamed, and blamed. They receive no justice. This compounds the trauma, because the victim not only suffers from the traumatic experience but also suffers the betrayal by the family and culture who didn't protect them or who ignored their pain. When harm is perpetrated by someone close in relationship, such as a family member, a study by Wills, Cuevas, and Sabina showed that the result is even greater psychological distress such as depression, anger, dissociation, and anxiety for the victim than if the perpetrator had been a stranger. We are most vulnerable to lasting harm when our family members hurt us, so the needs of the victim must always be at the center.

Creating a culture of accountability means that there must be consequences for those who harm others. Most victims of crime or abuse will never receive any semblance of justice from our criminal justice system. The alternative to the criminal justice system should not be nothing. We can create other avenues for helping victims find a sense of justice, and this can include holding family members who harm accountable. Their access to the family may be restricted until safety can be assessed. They must own up to what they have done and take accountability. They must engage in repair and make the necessary changes so that the abuse will no longer continue. We can support those who have harmed in learning to change their behaviors, and we can support those who have been harmed in their healing process by validating their experiences, asking what they need from us, and meeting those needs. This is a practice of community accountability, community healing, and generational transformation.

Reflection and deconstruction

★ How have you seen abuse or harm handled within your family, community, or culture? Does it work? Why or why not?

★ How would you structure a culture of accountability? What processes should be in place? What might victims need? What might those who harm need?

ESTABLISHING A RESOURCE

Your cultural heritage extends even further than your immediate family. Your cultural heritage is not a gift from only your parents or their parents or even their parents, but is a long legacy of ancestral gifts and tools. Sometimes when I work with clients who carry painful mother and father wounds, or have experienced harm within their family systems, we use an ancestral connection meditation to locate an ancestor we can draw from who doesn't carry these wounds. This serves as an important reminder that although we have generational trauma, we also have generational wisdom, healing, and well-being, and a family that extends for many generations back and forward. The practice, adapted from one I sat in led by Nir Esterman during the 2020 Embodied Trauma Conference, goes as follows...

If you would like to establish an ancestral resource, allow yourself to find a place of calm and quiet where you won't be disturbed. You may want to set up the space by making a comfortable place to sit, maybe lighting a candle, or playing soft music. Get into a comfortable spot with your eyes closed and allow your breath to flow gently. When you are ready, allow yourself to begin searching for an ancestral resource deep in your family line. Imagine in your mind's eye you are journeying back through the ancestors, through those who came before you. You may see those who struggled, had hardships, or experienced traumas you can still feel today. Allow yourself to journey until you meet someone who came before them. Journey back, even if it is just one generation before. Wherever it takes you is okay. Just go back through the generations until you find just one ancestor who was not affected by these systems, this oppression.

You don't have to know anything about them or what they look like. Simply allow some representation of them to come forward. They may come in their human form, or they may come as another representation, such as an image, a sensation, a color, or a flow of energy. Just notice them as they arrive.

You don't need to converse or interact with this ancestor. Simply notice their presence. Just know that at some point in time, in your ancestral line, there was once a human being who did not suffer from this trauma, or this self-doubt or identity confusion, or this shame that you feel now. There was someone once who felt more whole, and who felt satisfied that they were enough. And they are a part of you.

Imagine a long line. It could be three people long, it could be 500 people long—this is the line that connects you to this ancestor, this person who had strength or well-being or confidence, or some quality that you would like to have for yourself.

This ancestor has this quality just because they didn't have to live in the systems or traumas that the next generations experienced. They didn't experience the same shame or exclusion, so they are more integrated, more whole, more at peace. Allow yourself to simply be in their presence, noticing what it feels like to be in touch with them. And when you are ready to go, make sure to thank them for visiting you. When you're ready re-open your eyes, take some breaths, and look around your peaceful space, returning to the present moment.

Once you are done, allow for some quiet time as this experience integrates, and when you are ready, reflect using some of the questions below.

Reflection and deconstruction

★ What is it like to consider those in your lineage who were more whole or who existed before deep wounding occurred?

★ What sensations or emotions did you notice in their presence?

★ If you felt a positive presence with an ancestor, how can you maintain this connection?

Remember that there is a more healthy and complete state available to you in your collective unconscious, in your family collective, in your cultural collective. We can experience healing connection by connecting with our lineage.

Remember, you are the descendant of your ancestors. You are the product of their courage, their resilience. You are a product of their art, their dance, their music, their celebrations, their garden, their joy. You are the seed they planted,

knowing they wouldn't see you bloom, but they planted any-
way. This lives within you at every moment, and no one can
take it from you. You can revisit them when you need to be
reminded by using this practice.

To heal from soul wounds, we must embrace the gifts given
to us by our cultural heritage and use them with intention
towards integration of all parts of ourselves. As human beings,
we are in constant evolution, and growth through challenge is
one of the key strengths of Latinx people. Through struggle we
overcome and learn more about our capabilities, determination, and strength. We are not static. Evolution, accompanied
by an embrace of our Latinx identity and cultural gifts and
rooted in the love of the collective, moves us towards healing.
In this chrysalis we can become self-actualized, community
actualized. We learn to honor and accept ourselves, to care
for ourselves, to nurture our well-being, and to have a feeling
of belonging and cooperation towards a higher vision for the
liberation of all oppressed peoples.

CHAPTER 7

IMMIGRATION STORIES MATTER

WRITING YOUR IMMIGRATION *TESTIMONIO*

Have you ever written your family's immigration story? Telling our family immigration story, our *testimonio*, is a powerful way of taking control of our own cultural narrative. Our stories matter. Who we tell this story to, why we tell it, and how we tell it matters. Our voices become a tool for countering the dominant narratives that drive harsh public attitudes towards Latinxs and immigration.

The prevailing narratives around immigration influence the way migrants are treated in their receiving countries socially, legally, and politically. They also impact the way Latinx people are treated more generally. Despite Latinxs living in territories that are now the U.S. for longer than this country has existed, Latinx people are the ethnic group most associated with immigration and therefore they are treated like outsiders.

Predominant discourse is often far divorced from the reality of Latinx immigration, and its root causes. A 24-hour news cycle using terms such as "illegal invasion" and "migrant surge" is false and dangerous, not only because it acts as if migration occurs in a vacuum, but also because it increases false negative beliefs about people who migrate.

In 2015, a study by Shin, Leal, and Ellison found the most consistently significant factor in shaping a person's opinion about immigration restrictions was their attitude towards Latinxs. A person's belief in stereotypes about Latinxs, their disrespect towards our culture, and their discomfort in our presence mattered more than the substance of the immigration policies themselves. Attitude towards Latinxs mattered more than even the respondents' own economic situation or political affiliation. Opinions about immigration in this country run on anti-Latinx attitudes.

Most Americans live in a false reality when it comes to understanding immigration to the U.S., and why people must migrate in the first place. This false reality acts as a block to seeing migrants as human beings worthy of safety and compassion. It also allows the U.S. government to problematize immigration when it is politically convenient without admitting that much of the immigration we have seen is the direct result of American foreign policy and the U.S.'s imperialistic quest for world domination.

For too long, immigration discourse has been controlled by those who refuse to see migration as a frequent and often necessary part of the human experience. These stories are told by those who refuse to see the U.S.' role in triggering global instability that forces many to leave their homes. We cannot let them tell our stories because these stories are ours to tell.

Reflection and deconstruction

★ When does your immigration story begin? Who and what played a role in the decision to come to the U.S.?

★ How did you or your family members get to the U.S.? What was the journey like? (You may need to ask other members of your family to get a fuller picture.)

★ What qualities did this migration require of those who made the journey?

★ What was gained and what was lost for those who made

the journey? If you were born later, what have you lost and gained because of their decision?

★ If someone were to hear this story, what would they think of you and your family? What would you want them to see, know, and understand?

MIGRATION IS UNIVERSAL

Migration is a universal part of the human experience. People have migrated for as long as they have been on this planet. People cannot be controlled or stopped by lines drawn on a map when their ability to live safely hangs in the balance. As migration researcher Heidie Castañeda writes:

> Migration is part of what it is to be human, with population movements shaping the globe throughout the history of our species as a fundamental impulse to seek out better living conditions, whether that means safety and security, adequate resources, or a healthier environment.

The U.S. has seen its Latinx population grow significantly in the last century. From 1960 to 2020 the Latinx population in the U.S. went from 6.3 million to 62.1 million. In that same period, the number of Latinx people who were foreign born increased more than 20 times, going from less than 1 million to 20.2 million.

The reasons for such significant growth of the Latinx population in the U.S. are complex, but the role of the U.S. in creating the conditions that have forced migration from Latin America and the Caribbean cannot be ignored, especially when it comes to U.S. intervention in other countries, U.S. global economic policy, and U.S. immigration policy. Understanding these root causes shifts how we as Latinx people understand our place in the U.S. and shows us why migrants do not deserve to carry burdens of blame when they are pushed to move in response to global social, political, and economic circumstances far beyond their control.

THE COLD WAR: LATIN AMERICA BECOMES A U.S. BATTLEGROUND

The U.S. has a long and devious history of creating problems in other places, to benefit U.S. foreign and economic interests, and to secure their status as a world power. Throughout the Cold War with the Soviet Union, the U.S. used Latin America as a proxy to battle against the Soviet Union and the boogey man of communism. The Cold War started shortly after the end of World War II in the late 1940s and continued until 1991 when the Soviet Union dissolved. During this time, the U.S.' primary goal was to maintain the Western Hemisphere as a united front against the Soviets and to stop the spread of communism by any means necessary.

Historian John Coatsworth writes:

> In the slightly less than a hundred years, from 1898 to 1994, the U.S. government has intervened successfully to change governments in Latin America a total of at least 41 times. That amounts to once every 28 months for an entire century.

This is an enormous number when you think how profoundly unstable a country would become after having their duly elected government overthrown by an outside entity. The U.S. military, through CIA operations, economic influence, occupations, and military coups, purposefully disrupted Latin American countries they feared had become too leftist. They were motivated by fear that Latin American countries would become allies of the Soviet Union and implement socialist or communist policies to reduce the global power of capitalism.

The U.S. supported right-wing dictators, brutal military regimes, and authoritarian governments throughout Latin America and the Caribbean. In doing so, they unleashed genocidal violence and social upheaval, and inflicted extreme trauma that will ripple through several generations. The U.S. interfered with the right of citizens of sovereign nations to determine their own futures and choose their own leaders. They cut democracy off at the knees in countries that had already struggled to find their way in the years after colonization. This history of intervention set into motion political, social, and economic conditions that have pushed many to leave their home countries in search of greater peace and stability. Many came to realize that one of the best ways to protect themselves from living in a place where their government is overthrown by the U.S. military, is to move to the U.S.

Examples of U.S. intervention in Latin America
Guatemala

In 1954, President Eisenhower ordered the CIA to initiate a coup to force out democratically elected leftist President Jacobo Arbenz, who had attempted to redistribute land to peasants. The U.S. again backed military coups in 1963, 1982, and 1983. During the Guatemalan Civil War, lasting from 1960 to 1996, the U.S. continued to back the Guatemalan military as they perpetrated a genocide against the Indigenous population. The genocide targeted the Ixil Mayas; the Q'anjob'al and Chuj Mayas; the K'iche' Mayas of Joyabaj, Zacualpa, and Chiché; and the Achi Mayas. An estimated 200,000 were either killed or disappeared during that period, and 1.5 million people were displaced: 80% of the victims were Mayan. Despite knowing that the army and their paramilitary allies were massacring Indigenous villagers, the CIA continued to equip and train Guatemalan security forces and provided $33 million to the military as a part of their anti-communism policy during the Cold War, a detail reported by Douglas Farah in *The Washington Post*. The abuses of the civil war in Guatemala, including the role of the U.S., are detailed in the Report of the Commission for Historical Clarification named *Guatemala: Memory of Silence*. Later, U.S. intelligence documents were declassified that further revealed U.S. awareness of grave human rights abuses while continuing to offer support.

The Civil War led to a mass exodus of asylum seekers, with 400,000 Guatemalans fleeing to the U.S., Mexico, and Canada in that time.

With a legacy of political instability, and violent control by the military and landowning elites, Guatemala today continues to experience high levels of violence, insecurity, rural poverty, and inequality. These are the main drivers of migration to the U.S. from Guatemala. Migrants are often seeking economic opportunities, and fleeing extortion, crime victimization, and corruption. By 2010, people from Guatemala had become the fourth largest Latin American-born group in the U.S.

El Salvador

During the Salvadoran Civil War of 1979–1992, U.S.-trained paramilitary groups became a part of the country's right-wing death squad militia. The death squads were fascist groups, supporting the interests of the military, elites, and wealthy landowners in their fight against left-wing guerilla groups. Throughout the war there were gross human rights violations. Civilians were subjected to torture, mutilation, forced disappearance, extrajudicial killing, and mass rape. Targets of violence were often workers, peasants, human rights advocates, labor unionists, journalists, clergy members, and students. These abuses are detailed in *From madness to hope: The 12-year war in El Salvador: Report of the Commission on the Truth of El Salvador* commissioned by the United Nations.

During this period, the U.S. gave El Salvador substantial military aid, economic aid, advisors, and training. The U.S. provided over $4.5 billion to El Salvador during this period, with Cara McKinney, in her review of the war, stating that some estimate it was closer to $6 billion. Much of this aid went to the formation of the Rapid Deployment Infantry Battalions, the same groups identified by the UN Truth Commission as "the primary agents of war crimes." The war resulted in the deaths of at least 75,000 people.[1]

Sociologists Cecilia Menjívar and Andrea Gómez Cervantes for the Migration Policy Institute lay out a thorough review of how the civil war supported by the U.S. continued violence and drove migration. The U.S.-fueled war displaced 1 million Salvadorans, about one-fifth of their population at the time, both within the country and in neighboring countries. About a half million of those came to the U.S. The U.S. would not recognize them as refugees needing asylum, because this would have contradicted U.S. foreign policy support for the war. This left many Salvadorans undocumented and vulnerable to deportation until the U.S. included a provision in the 1990 Immigration Act that provided Temporary Protected Status (TPS).

The civil war left behind a militarized society steeped in both psychosocial trauma, extreme inequality, and a high number of weapons. Dr. Martín-Baró described the impact of the extreme violence of the war as creating a "militarization of the mind." The history of state violence left behind weak governance and low respect for democratic institutions. Most of the population are unable to earn enough to survive. This allows drug cartels and various organized-crime groups to recruit members needing opportunity, especially youth who have very few options. The boost in migration from the civil war has continued since the war, due to persistent violence.

Deportations of Salvadorans from the U.S. significantly aggravated violent trends in El Salvador. Deportees included young Salvadorans who, rejected by American society, had formed gangs in the U.S. The MS-13 gang was started in El

---

1   Ignacio Martín-Baró, to whom this book owes a debt of gratitude, was a social psychologist PhD and Jesuit priest living in El Salvador during the war. On November 16, 1989, he, along with seven others, was assassinated by U.S.-trained troops of the elite Atlacatl Battalion. His work focused on the liberation of the oppressed in Latin America, and he challenged the field of psychology to develop critical consciousness and a new praxis focused on the needs of the people. His work inspired the development of liberation psychology.

Salvador by Salvadorans deported from the U.S. Recently, levels of violence have been even higher than during wartime, resulting in the election of Nayib Bukele as president. He has cracked down on violence at the expense of maintaining civil liberties and the constitution. Ripple effects of the civil war continue to drive Salvadorans away from their homes and towards the U.S., seeking asylum.

In 1980, early in the war, the U.S. was home to 94,000 Salvadoran-born people. In the next ten years that number grew to over 700,000. Salvadorans are the third largest population of Latinx origin in the U.S., as of 2021, with a population of about 2.5 million, and the largest Central American group. From 2000 to 2021, the Salvadoran-origin population increased by 250%.

Chile

A staff report of the Select Committee to Study Governmental Operations with Respect to Intelligence Activities (United States Select Committee on Intelligence 1975) describes the U.S. Covert Action in Chile from 1963–1974.

1963–1974: The CIA made extensive efforts to destabilize Chile and influence their elections. The U.S. spent $13 million on covert action in Chile, attempting to influence their elections, including funding opposition political parties and aiding right-wing groups. In 1970, President Salvador Allende, head of the Popular Unity coalition including socialists, communists, radicals, and dissident Christian democrats, won in a narrow election. He began to institute socialist policies such as redistribution of land, free education and healthcare, and nationalization of banks and copper mines.

1973: The CIA secretly and without adequate government oversight supported the overthrow of democratically elected President Allende in a violent coup. This began the U.S.-backed military dictatorship of Augusto Pinochet, which lasted for 17 years. The coup marked an end to Chile's long tradition of constitutional government, and the beginning of one of the most brutal dictatorships in Latin American history. During Pinochet's reign, the military used repressive and violent acts, including forced exile, torture, summary execution, kidnapping, and unlawful detention, to create a climate of fear and control. The government tortured 40,000 people, killed more than 3000, and caused the disappearance of more than a thousand others. Hundreds of thousands were forced into exile. Victims included Indigenous peoples, Catholics, the rural community, former government officials, and members of leftist political parties. Pinochet, guided by a group of U.S.-educated Chilean economists, instituted neoliberal free-market policies which led them into an international debt crisis and the collapse of the Chilean economy by 1982.

Chilean immigration to the U.S. increased after 1990, with many leaving as political asylum seekers or refugees. Today, Chile continues to struggle with political, financial, and social inequality stemming from Pinochet's policies.

In other countries
During the Cold War, the U.S. used similar strategies as those described above to subvert democracy and influence politics in the Dominican Republic, Nicaragua, Panama, Bolivia, Argentina, Cuba, and Brazil. After the Cold War ended, the U.S. would continue to support coups, and other sorts of undemocratic political transitions, albeit with decreased fervor. As their place as the winner of the Cold War was solidified, the U.S. shifted away from military intervention as a means of control and towards the use of economic controls. But of course, old habits die hard, so in Haiti in 2004, Honduras in 2009, Paraguay in 2012, Brazil in 2016, and Bolivia in 2019, the U.S. again supported the overthrow of governments via military coup. The U.S. also supported attempted coups in Bolivia in 2008, Ecuador in 2010, and Venezuela in 2019.

The U.S. continues to use military coups to devastate target countries, knowing full well that these covert regime changes make the target country more likely to be thrown into civil war, threatening civilians with mass killings and decades of violence, poverty, and instability. This all makes it more likely that people will be forced out into neighboring countries as migrants and refugees.

NEOLIBERALISM AND ECONOMIC CONTROL

After the Cold War, the U.S. continued to prioritize its own geopolitical interests and those of multinational corporations over democracy, sovereignty, and the will of the people in Latin America and the Caribbean. The break-up of the Soviet Union meant that capitalism was now poised to become the dominant global economic system. The U.S. turned its attention towards its next mission—getting other countries to fall in line.

Around this time, Latin American countries were in precarious financial positions, which the U.S. immediately used to its advantage. In the 1980s, Mexico and other Latin American countries struggled to pay their debts to the U.S. and Europe. When Latin American nations went to powerful institutions like the World Bank and International Monetary Fund (IMF) for assistance, they were given loans but with strict conditions. To receive help, they had to agree to undertake broad economic reform, and shift to a set of free-market economic policies, often referred to as The Washington Consensus.

The Washington Consensus, a term coined by economist John Williamson in 1989, was a set of ten recommended policy prescriptions for improving economic performance. They included privatizing state-owned enterprises such as oil, gas, and transportation. They also suggested adopting free-trade policies, for instance reducing tariffs to make it cheaper for foreign companies to sell their goods in Latin America. They encouraged open markets with little to no government regulation. The goal of The Washington Consensus was to attract foreign investment while decreasing government control over the economy. In exchange for adopting these policies, the

foreign lenders like the IMF moved the high interest external debts of some Latin American countries into long-term
bonds, which made the payments more manageable for Latin
American countries, although the debt continued to increase.
The U.S. used the IMF to force Latin American and the
Caribbean to end a period where they had heavily focused on
nationalism, state-owned industries like gas and oil, domestic manufacturing, and government protection of domestic
industries against foreign competition. These were policies
designed to reduce Latin America's reliance on imports, and
to decrease its dependence on the more powerful countries.
The result of these neoliberal policies, described in Mark
Weisbrot's book *Failed*, was that "for more than 20 years during the neoliberal era, Latin America suffered a collapse of
economic growth that was unprecedented in the region for
at least a century, and indeed uncommon in the history of
modern capitalism." Economic interventions such as these
again created conditions where people were forced to leave
their homes.

UNINTENDED CONSEQUENCES: THE NORTH AMERICAN FREE TRADE AGREEMENT (NAFTA) AND THE ERA OF GLOBALIZATION

Sin maiz, no hay pais. (Without corn, there is no country.)

—MEXICAN PROTEST SLOGAN AND NAME OF FOOD
SOVEREIGNTY CAMPAIGN THAT FIGHTS AGAINST
THE USE OF GMO CROPS IN MEXICO

To see how neoliberalism has worked out we can look to
Mexico, and the adoption of the North American Free
Trade Agreement (NAFTA). NAFTA is a telling example of
the impact of neoliberalism on a country, and the vast unintended consequences regarding immigration. NAFTA was a
landmark trade deal between the U.S., Canada, and Mexico
that came into effect in 1994. It was signed into law by Bill

Clinton, although seeds of the bill were planted by Ronald Reagan during his administration. The bill received bipartisan support in Congress.

NAFTA created a free-trade zone between the three countries by eliminating tariffs and trade restrictions, allowing for the free flow of capital and goods. The capitalist dream of open markets was further realized. NAFTA allowed corporations to move production into Mexico where labor was cheaper, and easily sell these cheaply made goods throughout the trade zone. NAFTA was touted as a first step to an eventual free-trade zone that would include not only the rest of Latin America but would encompass the Western Hemisphere.

Michael Wilson, the director of the Heritage Foundation, a powerful Christian conservative thinktank, in 1993 called NAFTA "Ronald Reagan's vision realized" and stated:

> NAFTA thus guarantees that American workers will remain the most competitive in the world and that American consumers will continue to have access to the world's finest goods and services...it will create an estimated 200,000 new jobs for Americans, reduce illegal immigration from Mexico, help tackle drug trafficking, strengthen Mexican democracy and human rights, and serve as a model for the rest of the world.

Proponents of the bill in Mexico had similar expectations. Mexico's then President Carlos Salinas de Gortari said NAFTA would modernize the Mexican economy, improve quality of life, and provide enough well-paying jobs that Mexicans would no longer need to travel to the U.S. to find work. As journalist Alejandro Portes stated, "It was supposed to be the magic wand."

To be allowed into NAFTA, President Salinas was required to make changes to the Mexican Constitution. The Salinas government reformed Article 27, which was a product of the hard-fought Mexican Revolution that allowed for Indigenous models of land sharing. Article 27 redistributed land, granting peasant subsistence farmers *ejidos*, which were communal plots of land owned by the collective community and not by any one individual. By reforming Article 27, the Salinas government ended the revolutionary commitment to land redistribution and ceased to recognize rights to socially or collectively titled land. Instead, they broke up communal land, allowing it to be bought and sold, and exploited for profit. The reforms disrupted deeply rooted Indigenous and peasant cultures.[2]

NAFTA was a success for large transnational corporations, which profited from cheap labor, deregulation, and borders open to the flow of goods and capital. NAFTA gave the middle class in Mexico access to an increased variety of cheap consumer goods. But it also had many unintended consequences and failed to live up to too many of its promises.

Mexico did not experience the economic growth that it expected after NAFTA, and unemployment worsened in the years after signing. NAFTA allowed American agri-business to flood the Mexican market with cheap corn, something Mexico had previously only imported when its own production wasn't enough to meet their needs. Now U.S. companies that received government subsidies allowing them to price their corn under production cost competed in the market with small-scale Mexican farmers. These Mexican farmers were no match for the subsidized Goliath corporate farms of the north, especially as they simultaneously lost government assistance they had relied on for survival.

According to Public Citizen, a nonprofit consumer advocacy organization, the price paid to Mexican farmers for corn fell by 66%, forcing many to abandon farming. Those who had debt on their land were unable to make their payments. Their land was quickly scooped up by agri-businesses, which, due

---

2   On January 1, 1994, the day NAFTA began, the Ejército Zapatista de Liberación, or Zapatista Army of National Liberation (EZLN), engaged in an armed uprising and released a manifesto to protest neoliberalism and oppression of the Indigenous population. The army was made up almost entirely of Indigenous people, and one-third women. The EZLN are from Chiapas, where their fight against the Mexican government and capitalism continues today.

to land reforms, were now allowed to buy peasant land. From 1991 to 2007, over two million Mexican farmers and farm-laborers were driven out of work. Small and medium-sized businesses in Mexico also took a huge hit, with an estimated 28,000 destroyed in NAFTA's first four years. These Mexican-owned businesses couldn't compete with American corporations selling cheap goods imported from Asia.

As Mexico experienced an unemployment crisis, many workers were forced into the informal job economy doing things like washing windows at a traffic stop or selling tamales on a street corner to make a living. They also experienced a huge surge in the price of consumer goods. In 2003, on the ten-year anniversary of NAFTA, *The Washington Post* reported that "19 million more Mexicans are living in poverty than 20 years ago...nearly one in every four Mexicans...are classified as extremely poor and unable to afford adequate food."

As agricultural and industrial workers in Mexico lost their jobs, they had no choice but to head north in search of work. They did so in greater numbers than before NAFTA, upending NAFTA's promise to curb Mexican immigration. During NAFTA's first six years, the number of annual immigrants from Mexico more than doubled. In some areas, formerly bustling cities became ghost towns, with all able adults going abroad in search of work. Families were separated as one or both parents had to leave in the hope of being able to earn enough elsewhere to provide for their children.

As workers traveled north, the majority undocumented, cities in the U.S. that had never had a large Latinx population before found their numbers increasing. Places like Georgia and North Carolina saw an increased presence of undocumented workers. The American media went on a smear campaign, calling these migrants dehumanizing names like "illegals" and screaming that Latinx migrants were stealing jobs from hardworking Americans. Never did they stop long enough to consider how and why these migration patterns were set in motion. Now, nearly three decades later we can clearly see that NAFTA not only failed to deliver on its promises, but in regard to immigration had the opposite intended effect.

Other countries in Latin America felt similar effects of the neoliberal policy shift. Brazil, Chile, and Argentina each embraced neoliberal policies and invited foreign investment and corporations into their countries. As in Mexico, the middle classes benefitted from neoliberal policies through access to more products like video recorders and cars, satellite TV, and fast-food chains. But also as in Mexico, the poor were left behind as poverty and inequality got worse, and social programs were taken away. The free market often ignores low-income markets, and there is little incentive to provide for the needs of the poor. As many lost jobs, their basic goods like rice, water, and telephone, now privatized, became more and more expensive.

By the 2000s, Latin American economies were imploding. In 2001, Argentina, a country that had followed all IMF instructions, defaulted on its foreign debts, and was thrown into an economic, political, and social crisis. Brazil saw a lack of economic growth, higher inequality, and an increase in violent crime. Countries soured to the promises of neoliberalism. As the Latin American public began to turn away from neoliberalism, they started to elect leaders who took a stand against these policies and called for reinvestment in society. Brazilians elected Luiz Inácio da Silva, "Lula," a former union leader, to the presidency. Bolivia elected Evo Morales, an Indigenous Aymara farmer in 2006. That same year Chile elected Michelle Bachelet, a socialist. In 2018, Mexico elected its first left-wing president in over three decades. Each of these new presidents endorsed a return to nationalism, programs for the poor, and resistance to domination by the U.S.

UNINTENDED CONSEQUENCES OF THE U.S. IMMIGRATION POLICY

The final piece to the often-disregarded influences on immigration is to explore the unintended consequences of the U.S.'

own immigration policy. Unexpectedly, changes in policy that were designed to be more restrictive instead led to significant increases in the Latinx population in the U.S.

The year 1965 represents a major turning point in immigration, the year the U.S. made amendments to the Immigration and Nationality Act. It repealed national origins quotas and replaced them with a new system that imposed a cap on visas for immigrants from the Western Hemisphere at 120,000. The new legislation also allowed citizens, often immigrants who naturalized, to sponsor their relatives to come to the U.S. This process called chain migration allowed many Latinx people to come to the U.S. Out of 33 million immigrants admitted to the U.S. from 1981 to 2016, about 20 million were chain-migration immigrants. Mexico has the highest rate of chain migration to the U.S.

The end of the *Bracero* program also occurred in 1965. This program allowed Mexican workers, about 450,000 annually, to enter the U.S. legally and temporarily to meet labor shortages. Migrants flowed legally between Mexico and the U.S. from the beginning of the program in 1942 until it was ended by Congress in 1964. In its 22 years, the *Bracero* program allowed 4.5 million Mexicans to work legally in the U.S. and then return home.

The established pattern of migration between Mexico and the U.S. at this time was circular with workers coming in to fill labor gaps, and then returning home. Ending the *Bracero* program didn't end the long-established flow of migrant workers, it just no longer offered the workers authorization. The changes to immigration policy no longer allowed for guest-worker visas and significantly capped permanent resident visas, meaning there was now no legal recourse available to the same flow of labor that had existed for decades. The U.S. and Mexico are closely connected economically so the need for labor didn't vanish. It is just that the same labor force was now considered illegal.

What was true before 1965 continued to be true afterwards, and today—the U.S. needs immigrant labor. In 2022, the U.S. Labor Department reported that there were almost twice as many job openings as unemployed workers. With the U.S. population aging, and labor force participation declining since the 1990s, the U.S. depends on immigrant labor to meet this demand. The U.S. economy functions due to immigrant labor. If that labor need is there, immigrants meet it.

The U.S. reliance on immigrants is rarely ever addressed in politics or media; instead they are villainized. After the end of the *Bracero* program, politicians grabbed onto this new supposed increase in illegal immigration because it was politically advantageous. It allowed them to demonize immigrants from Mexico and Latin America to stoke fear and increase their own base of support. In the late 1960s, the media began to describe this increase in illegal immigration as a national crisis, despite it being the same flow of labor that had existed and not bothered them before 1965. A narrative where Latinx people are seen as a threat wasn't anything new. This story quickly grew in popularity allowing for the passage of increasingly restrictive immigration policies, and more focus on enforcement actions. More funding went to the Immigration and Naturalization Service and later to Immigration and Custom Enforcement (ICE) and Customs and Border Protection.

The changes to policy and funding, supported by the media frenzy, led to an increase in border apprehensions. The increase in border apprehensions was used to fuel the narrative that the country was under invasion. This creates a revolving door cycle that has been described as a self-feeding chain divorced from the reality. In the 1970s the flow of undocumented migrants had actually stabilized, and in the late 1980s and early 90s illegal immigration actually dropped. However, due to these new policies, the number of arrests and deportations drastically increased even while illegal immigration was coming down.

According to Office of Homeland Security Statistics, prior to the mid-1990s, annual deportations had been under 50,000 for decades. These numbers began to change starting in 1996, when almost 70,000 were deported. Year after year these numbers rose drastically. In the year 2000, over 188,000 were deported. Deportations peaked in 2013 with 432,228. These numbers were more fuel to support the invasion narrative, and after 9/11 the narratives took on a tone beyond posing migrants as a threat to American jobs but now positing that migrants were a threat to national security.

A major unintended consequence of the changes in immigration policy and enforcement was the increase in the number of undocumented migrants in the U.S. Because there was increased enforcement at the borders, fewer people returned home after working as they had done during the *Bracero* program. People began to stay because multiple border crossings became increasingly risky, and increasingly expensive. The longer they stayed, the more likely they were to eventually send for their loved ones to join them in the U.S. What had once been a population of temporary male migrant workers became a settled population of families. A sharp decline in outflow of unauthorized migrants, and stable inflow of unauthorized migrants, resulted in the growth of the undocumented population.

The narratives around immigration to the U.S. often frame the country as under siege by migrants from other countries who choose to come here purely for their own benefit. What is often ignored is the U.S. role in forcing those migrations, and the U.S. reliance on this stream of workers to meet labor needs. Over time, the U.S. has had increasingly restrictive immigration policy and enforcement, but these changes have failed to reduce the flow of migrants to the U.S. What they have accomplished is a drastically reduced outflow of immigrants. And the longer people stay, they more likely they are to settle long term. Without education regarding the true factors that influence migration it is easy to get swept up into the dominant narratives where immigrants are demonized in the media and public consciousness. Immigrants are made scapegoats for U.S. government policy decisions. There is a lot more to the story than we are told, which is why we Latinxs must be the ones to tell it.

Latinxs have been made the face of immigration in the U.S. It is time we took control of the narrative, speak truth to power, and know that while many people do come here to make a better life, they often do so because their chances to do that at home were destroyed by coups and corporations.

Reflection and deconstruction

★ Did U.S. intervention play a role in you, your family, or people like you leaving home?

★ How were your people treated when they arrived in the U.S.? Why do you think that is?

★ Did your family plan to stay in the U.S.?

★ Has this information impacted your views on immigration?

★ Does this change how you tell your own family migration story?

CHAPTER 8

TWICE AS PERFECT

I didn't find freedom in assimilation because there is no freedom in racist ideas.

—JULISSA ARCE, *YOU SOUND LIKE A WHITE GIRL*

In the iconic movie *Selena* there is a well-known scene that nearly every Latinx person living in the U.S. can relate to at some point in their lives.

Selena and her brother, played by Jennifer Lopez and Jacob Vargas, are riding in a van with their father Abraham, played by the legendary Edward James Olmos. The siblings are trying to convince him to accept an invitation to play in Monterrey, Mexico.

Abraham tells them they are not ready to play for a Mexican audience. He says that although Selena can sing perfectly in Spanish, she does not speak Spanish perfectly. "The press will eat you up," Abraham cautions. He goes on to explain:

Being Mexican American is tough. Anglos jump all over you if you don't speak English perfectly. Mexicans jump all over you if you don't speak Spanish perfectly... We got to be twice as perfect as everybody else! ... We got to be more Mexican than the Mexicans and more American than Americans but at the same time. It's exhausting!

This scene always elicits knowing laughter and enthusiastic

nods of agreement from a Latinx audience. And if you pay attention a little longer you may also notice some twinges of resentment or frustration as the audience is reminded of the impossible paradox that we find ourselves in—to be twice as perfect. As Latinx people in the U.S., we know all too well the pressures of living between two cultures, and not quite feeling at home in either. We know the feeling of being looked down on by white Americans for not being white, and we also know the painful sting of not being accepted by our own people.

ACCULTURATIVE STRESS: *NI DE AQUÍ, NI DE ALLÁ* (NEITHER FROM HERE NOR FROM THERE)

In our community we often use the saying *ni de aquí, ni de allá* to describe what the mental health field calls acculturation. Acculturation describes the ways immigrant or minority individuals or groups adopt cultural features from the mainstream culture. People acculturate to different degrees, with some favoring their Latinx culture more strongly, some favoring dominant American culture more strongly, and others trying to find a balance between the two. Assimilation, the process of fully adopting the mainstream culture and losing your native culture, is one potential outcome of acculturation.

Acculturation happens no matter what to some degree. But what we don't often realize is the true cost of this process for our emotional, spiritual, and even physical well-being. In the mental health field, the distress one feels while trying to integrate two different cultures is called acculturative stress. Acculturative stress happens because we are simultaneously navigating two different cultures with conflicting expecta- tions. How I talk, what language I speak, how I behave, and how I present myself can all shift depending on whether I find myself in a more Latinx dominant or American white suprem- acy culture dominant space, or somewhere in between. This ability to shift between spaces is a skill we develop over time; however, just because we're good at something doesn't mean it's good for us.

Considering how important culture is to our lives, acculturation can present a difficult problem. Culture shapes values and expectations. Culture influences the way we interact with others, what we eat, how we dance, and the way we raise our children. When we have one foot in one culture and the other foot in a different culture, each asking us to value and prioritize different things, we can again feel split apart. Acculturative stress leaves us overwhelmed, and often feeling stretched thin.

The collectivist values of our Latinx culture and the individualism demanded by American culture want opposite things from us. Our Latinx culture asks us to value family and community, and to think of others before ourselves. It asks us to support our family members when they need us, to slow down and spend time with them. Our culture also asks us to make our family members' sacrifices for us worthwhile by becoming successful. Our Latinx culture guides us to connect to what we hold sacred, to feel the energies of the universe, and to be open to the forces of life even when we don't quite understand them.

American culture, on the other hand, tells us to be rational and scientific, that time is money, and that life is a competition. It tells us that our value is measured by how much money we make and how much we work. American culture tells us to pull ourselves up by our bootstraps, because everyone is responsible for themselves. It says we don't owe others anything and that nothing is owed to us. Dominant American culture sees dependence on others as a problem, and even a sign of being unwell. It demands a rugged individualism with a promise that success will feel sweet when you can proclaim, "I did this on my own."

How could anyone possibly satisfy these two different cultures at the same time? What wins in one, loses in the other. Without the recognition of the enormous difficulty of this task we start to feel as if we're failing, letting those around us down, or as if we just aren't good enough. We need perspective to realize what a difficult task we've been given. No one ever slows us down and says, "You know, you don't have to please everyone, right?" Living both inside and outside Latinx and American cultures is hard.

Acculturative stress can be made worse when it creates family conflict. Not all members in a family will integrate Latinx culture and American culture in the same way or at the same rate. How one acculturates depends a lot on what spaces they spend time in, and who they are around. A new immigrant from Venezuela, who moves to a community where other Venezuelan or Latinx immigrants live, who finds a job where they work with other Latinx Spanish speakers, will be more likely to maintain their culture. That same person's child, however, can have quite a different experience. They will go to school where they are exposed to the dominant American culture's history, art, and literature. They will be taught to value the U.S., and that the U.S. is the world leader of freedom and democracy. Nearly every famous historical figure they will learn about will be a white male. They will do the pledge of allegiance and learn English. English will be associated with success. This environment will speed up acculturation, and American culture will be integrated for this kid in a much different way than for their parent.

Sometimes parents and family members see signs of acculturation in their children and perceive this to be willful defiance or a full-out rejection of the family's culture. A child growing up in the U.S. may be taught at school to be assertive and direct, to raise their hand, and give their opinion. This same behavior at home can be seen as disrespectful. Parents may not appreciate just how much influence the world outside the family can have on their child.

When families have acculturative conflicts both sides can feel misunderstood and rejected by their loved ones. This mis-understanding can create distance between family members as each person sees the other as pushing them away. To feel rejected by our family or community for our accommodations to American culture causes great sadness for many. A study study by Carly Thornhill and colleagues on intergenerational conflicts found that family conflicts due to differences in values, expectations, and acculturation levels led to depression and low self-esteem for Latinx college students.

When our families lose their cohesion, it can weaken one of our greatest forms of protection, a strong connection with our Latinx identity. Parents, fearing their child is losing their culture, may become even more strict, controlling, or traditional in their expectations which can make the situation worse. Kids and their parents feel the push/pull of each culture.

Parents may not also realize how their child's integration of American culture is a tool not just for their own survival, but for the survival of the family. The children of Latinx immigrants often become translators, and not just linguistic translators, but also cultural translators, helping each to understand the other. This is especially the case when their families have limited economic resources, or their parents didn't receive adequate education in their home country. First-generation Latinxs become the connection point between their parents and the dominant society. Many have found themselves doing things like translating tax forms, rental agreements, job applications, and even their own report cards to their parents. They recall being at doctors' appointments trying to guess the correct English or Spanish word for a medical term, body part, or ailment. As one of my students said during a lecture on this topic, "Have you ever had to ask your mom if she's sexually active?" This is the space many Latinx first-generation people find themselves inhabiting.

For first-generation Latinxs, the job of translator often started at young ages where the size of the job was greater than their current social or emotional maturity, but out of necessity they figured it out. Because of the pressure on first-generation kids to help their families, they learn the ins and outs of American culture that much faster. They also often learn they must be brave in uncomfortable situations and be adaptive problem-solvers without having someone to ask for help. This can create a strong, sometimes problematic, sense of responsibility. Sometimes they learn to fake it as best they can, not wanting to let their parents down, and setting the stage for a future of having difficulty saying no or asking others for help. They do their best to not only understand what the world needs from their family, but also how to explain that to their parents.

Reflection and deconstruction

★ Have you ever felt the pressure of acculturative stress? If so, what has it been like for you?

★ What elements of Latinx culture do you want to preserve and maintain as a part of your personal culture?

★ What elements of American culture have you accepted or taken on?

★ How has acculturation impacted your relationships with other Latinx people?

NO SABO: LANGUAGE LOSS AND LATINX IDENTITY

A major point of contention in our community is around language. Some think that speaking Spanish is synonymous with being Latinx, often forgetting that Brazilians speak Portuguese. As a result, there are many Latinx people who feel less than because they do not speak Spanish fluently, or at all. The term "*no-sabo* kid" is often used to make fun of Latinx people who do not speak Spanish, and answer with the incorrect phrase *no sabo* instead of *no sé*, for "I don't know."

Spanish is heavily associated with our cultural heritage, although it is of course deeply intertwined with colonialism. Nevertheless, not speaking Spanish can be seen as a rejection of one's cultural identity or a sign of assimilation. What many fail to consider is just how difficult it can be to maintain fluency in a second language, especially when facing language discrimination on one side and judgment for how well you speak it on the other. Many families struggle to maintain fluency in Spanish or Portuguese over the generations, and it is not for lack of trying.

The field of linguistics has long known about the three-generation process of language loss. It was first observed in the large wave of European immigrants who arrived in the late 1800s and has continued in the Latinx and Asian immigrants who have arrived since the mid-1960s. This loss occurs because immigrants to the U.S., who may or may not learn English, will usually prefer to speak their native language at home with their families. Their children will become bilingual. Their parents' native tongue is their home language, and English is used outside the home. Despite this second generation being bilingual, sociolinguistics research has found that they will likely prefer to speak in English and use this language more often. When they have their own children, they tend to speak English in their homes. This means the grandchildren of immigrants are very likely to be monolingual English speakers, with little knowledge of their grandparents' language. They will have been raised in English-speaking homes and live in an English-speaking world. They may still be exposed to their families' native language through time spent with their grandparents or even in their communities, but that often won't be enough to fully learn the native language.

Our Latinx communities have not been saved from this three-generation process. One study found that by the third generation, three-fourths of Cuban children and two-thirds of Mexican children spoke only English. Overall, the number of Latinx people who speak Spanish at home has declined. The Pew Research Center found that in the year 2000, 78% of Latinx people spoke Spanish at home, and by 2021 that number was down to 68%. For U.S.-born Latinxs, that number went from 66% to 55%.

Not speaking Spanish or Portuguese can be a major reason Latinx people who live in the U.S. feel they are not fully a part of the Latinx culture. They are often blamed for not knowing the language. People's assumption around language is often that if your parents speak another language, you will be exposed to it frequently, and that just this exposure should be enough for you to learn it too. Unfortunately, it just isn't that easy. Teaching your child a second language requires balanced exposure to both languages, which would mean hearing, reading, and talking in just as much Spanish or Portuguese as English. It also requires opportunities to interact with multiple different speakers—not an easy thing to do without significant effort and intention on behalf of the parents, and even then, it isn't a guarantee as the child ages and spends more time with peers or out of the home. When you combine this with the fact that the Spanish language is looked down on in the U.S., and Spanish language speakers have been punished and discriminated against, it is clear that many of us don't get a fair opportunity to learn.

Reflection and deconstruction

★ What is your language story?

★ What is your relationship to your family or ancestors' native language? Has this impacted your life or sense of cultural connection?

THE LATINX HEALTH PARADOX

Despite having less access to healthcare resources, among other disadvantages, Latinx immigrants to the U.S., even those who are poor, have better health outcomes than those born in the U.S., as demonstrated by a multitude of research studies such as the one led by L. Franzini. The longer a Latinx person lives in the U.S., the worse their health outcomes are. This phenomenon is called the immigrant paradox or, more specifically, the Latinx health paradox. In fact, a public health study led by Clara Barajas found that even when controlling for healthcare access and utilization, the paradox was maintained.

The paradox also applies to risky behaviors such as alcohol and substance use. A study by Guadalupe Bacio, Vickie Mays, and Anna Lau (2013) found that being a U.S. born Latinx teen puts you at greater risk for alcohol use compared to immigrant adolescents. They also found that teens whose parents were U.S. born are more likely to experience alcohol-related problems than adolescents whose parents were born elsewhere.

Longer lengths of time living in the U.S. was found to be significantly related to lower self-esteem among Latino adolescents in a study led by Paul Smokowski (2010), while Marysue Heilemann and colleagues (2002) found that women who spent their childhood in Mexico had less depression and more life satisfaction than their peers who spent time in the U.S. during childhood.

In fact, Stanley Sue and June Chu (2003), in their review of minority mental health data, found that Mexican Americans born outside the U.S. have better mental health outcomes than those who were born in the U.S., and even better mental health than white people in the U.S.

Latinx people who speak only English have been shown to have some of the worst severity of mental health conditions of the Latinx population. Being born in the U.S. places us at higher risk for depression, anxiety, and, most significantly, alcohol and substance abuse.

A contributor to these negative mental and physical health outcomes is the level of acculturation and acculturative stress. A meta-analysis by Eunju Yoon and colleagues (2013) found that a higher level of acculturation is a factor in negative mental health outcomes. Acculturative stress is linked to increased mental health issues, such as depression, anxiety, and psychological stress. Our mental and physical health worsen as we adopt more dominant American lifestyles and values and move further from our own culture.

For Latinxs born in the U.S., the acculturative stress begins the day they are born, which provides some understanding to the Latinx health paradox. Stress is toxic to all systems of the body, and when it is experienced on a chronic basis the effects accumulate, leading to more severe health outcomes. Those who immigrate begin their exposure to this specific type of acculturative stress later in life, giving them some protection. For those born in the U.S., acculturative stress begins to accumulate from day one and is present during significant developmental periods in their life like childhood. This, paired with stigma regarding mental health care, can mean we don't get the support we need when we need it. When we add in the fact that finding a mental health provider who understands the challenges of living between American and Latinx culture is not an easy task, we can see why this remains so pervasive.

Some might think that achieving "success" in the U.S. could help us get around the paradox and find our way back to feeling healthy and well. Unfortunately, it can put you at higher risk for mistreatment. A 2023 study by social work researchers Chiara Sabina and colleagues found that economic advancement increased the risk of being the victim of a hate crime, and of discrimination, harassment, microaggressions, and other types of crimes that result from bias against Latinxs. The researchers found that when a Latinx person is more acculturated and they experience upward mobility, they find themselves in spaces with people who find them threatening and treat them as such. Because they are more acculturated, they are also more able to pick up on the nuances of racist behaviour, such as microaggressions, than a less acculturated Latinx person would. Violent discrimination is often used to remind this successful Latinx person that even though they have achieved some "success" they are still subordinate. When a person has high levels of acculturation, but also has a strong sense of their Latinx identity and Latinx pride, they can tolerate these stressors better. However, when a person is highly acculturated and less connected to their Latinx identity, the research shows they are more likely to suffer and experience mental health disorders.

Many Latinx people who work hard to get an education and find themselves in professional job roles struggle with the negative experiences they are exposed to. One study on

Latinas physicians and medical students led by Gabriella Geiger found that 54.5% of the Latinas surveyed reported negative ethnicity-based interactions from patients and/or patients' families and 71.8%, from others in the medical field. The women reported high rates of depression (76.2%) and anxiety (92.6%). Many of the women struggled to feel a sense of belonging and being good enough, with over 90% reporting experiencing imposter syndrome.

It isn't that we as Latinx people are not competent, good enough, or don't belong, it is that we don't fit into the white supremacist culture's expected image of a professional, so these spaces try to push us out.

When a person has high levels of acculturation, but also a strong sense of their Latinx identity and Latinx pride, they can tolerate these stressors better. Research by Krysia Mossakowski on ethnic identity found that a strong ethnic identity buffers against the stress of racial and ethnic discrimination. A study led by Esther Calzada on Mexican-origin mothers found that strong ethnic identity also protects against depression. However, when a person is highly acculturated and less connected to their Latinx identity, the research shows they are more likely to experience mental health disorders.

TO ASSIMILATE OR NOT?

It is easy to see why acculturation and eventually full assimilation would be encouraged for Latinx immigrants. After all, how can you achieve the American Dream if you don't become American first? Since the early 1900s, the American ethos has promoted the idea of the U.S. as a melting pot for different cultures and people. There is an assumption that people from other countries who move to the U.S. will blend into the melting pot, and eventually lose their cultural distinctiveness to become simply American. American mythology says that all Americans are equal so the idea of becoming one sounds very enticing. But history has shown us that the U.S. has not been able to live up to the promise of all citizens being equal under the law, and the melting pot doesn't hold true for all immigrants.

The idea of the U.S. as a melting pot began when a wave of European immigrants, about 18 million people between 1890 and 1920, were absorbed into American society. These immigrants came from places like Ireland, Germany, and Italy. Over the generations they mostly lost direct ties to their cultural heritage. As they were brought into the American mainstream culture, they were no longer seen as Irish or German, they became Americans. But it is important to say that they were also allowed to become Americans. Today their descendants would largely be considered white and receive the many unearned privileges that come with that racial identification. Their Americanness will not be called into question.

In a highly racialized society like the U.S., Black and brown Latinx folks are not given the same opportunity to be seen as fully American. Our features will always signal an otherness, even if we learn to take on the dominant white culture's values, traditions, beliefs, and expectations. We'll still get the famous question, "Where are you from?" And even for those of us born in the U.S who can say, "I'm from here" we know to be ready for the automatic follow-up, "Oh...where are your parents from?" To be viewed as Latinx in the U.S. is nearly synonymous with being seen as an immigrant, an outsider. Being on the receiving end of this question is a sign that the narrative of the U.S. as a melting pot doesn't hold true. Some things don't melt while other parts of ourselves we refuse to lose to the sauce.

White supremacy culture plays a significant role in acculturation processes. When we think about the ways we learn dominant American culture we consider things like school, TV, movies, relationships, and other direct exposures to the mainstream. We often overlook how things such as daily microaggressions including passive insults or sly invalidations, or other racial traumas are also the mediums of acculturation. We learn what is expected of us in dominant society from the responses we get from others.

Getting picked on at school because your homemade lunch is different, your clothes are different, you speak differently, you wear gold jewelry, or because you have hair on your arms tells you a lot about what people like and don't like. So does your teacher automatically saying to you, "Tell your mother that..." while she stands beside you, because just by the look of her the teacher assumes she can't speak English. This teaches us just as much about what's expected of us as the day's American history lesson.

Psychologist William Ming Liu and colleagues write that acculturation is a "continuing process wherein some people of color learn explicitly via racism, microaggressions, and racial trauma about their racial positionality; White racial space; and how they're supposed to accommodate White people's needs, status, and emotions." Liu and his colleagues go on to say that the acculturation process in and of itself is a form of racial trauma, and a product of living in a white supremacist place and culture.

When Latinx people are exposed to microaggressions and racism, we are both directly and indirectly being told how to behave around white people. When white people or their proxies enact these racial aggressions towards us, they are trying to remind us that they own that space, and that we are visitors. We learn to make accommodations to white expectations, but instead it's called politeness, social etiquette, professionalism, or code-switching. This allows some of us to fit into white spaces, and even thrive in these white spaces if we can get good at it. We know how to adjust ourselves to avoid tension or outright hostility, and to allow white people to feel comfortable. It often involves being smaller, quieter, and more subdued.

Many Latinx and other people of color know not to speak their native language to each other around white people for risk of being accused of gossiping about them or of being rude. A more hostile group might mutter, "This is America, we speak English." We learn to make white people comfortable. We, however, are left to deal with the resulting feeling that we aren't being our true selves.

Dr. María Lugones was a feminist philosopher from Argentina. She described the experience of being an outsider in the mainstream white culture as "'world'-traveling," a skill where one knows how to go into the worlds of the mainstream, and then back to worlds where we feel more at home. Dr. Lugones found that this practice was a necessary, and often compulsory, survival skill. We have no choice but to enter hostile white worlds. Within these worlds, we might use our knowledge of the language and norms to appear at ease in that world. Because we know what it is like to inhabit different worlds, and travel between them, we have a unique and more nuanced perspective of ourselves and others. We can observe each world, and ourselves within them. We can observe ourselves, not as a static being, but as having different versions of self. We can see the absurdity of some aspects of each world. We can hold complexity. And we can do this in a way that those who only know the dominant culture cannot.

In my work with clients, we are often focused on recognizing and harnessing our many strengths, gifts, and powers. Sometimes this means coming into a place of being able to control what was once automatic, making the subconscious conscious. When we find ourselves code-switching between spaces, but we don't understand what it is or why we do it, it can feel unsettling. Sometimes we interpret this as lacking a true sense of self, or we judge ourselves for pandering to whiteness, as if we're betraying who we are or where we come from. But I challenge you to look beyond that, to see this as a unique skill, and to use this to your advantage. The catch is to not allow yourself to be deceived and confused about which world is yours; to not surrender to the dominant culture and assimilate. When we lose ourselves to assimilation, to whiteness, we suffer greatly. When we stay in touch with our true core, our culture, and allow world-traveling to be a skill used with intention, we are more powerful.

When we use this skillset, but also maintain our roots, our cultural pride, we can bring more of our true self into whatever world we inhabit. We go from trying to fit ourselves into the mold of what whiteness expects of a person, a teacher, a politician, and so on, to leading with our core self and showing the world how a Latinx person lives, thrives, teaches, or leads. Understanding the systems at play, and how threats to whiteness are treated, it is also important to know that our ways won't be rewarded by the system, because the system wants one thing—adherence to white culture. And that's okay. We do this for ourselves, our families, and people like us. Our daily living is a form of resistance.

Reflection and deconstruction

★ Have you experienced microaggressions, race-based invalidations or insults, or other forms of racial trauma? How did this impact you? What did it teach you?

★ How do you feel when you are in majority white spaces? Do you make any accommodations to how you act, dress, talk, or behave? Why or why not?

★ When or where do you feel most like your true self? Are you a "'world' traveler"? What has that been like?

★ What strengths come from being able to navigate different cultural spaces? What challenges come from it? What would you like to keep doing? What would you like to do differently?

CHAPTER 9

FINDING HEALTHY COLLECTIVISM

Balance, Setting Boundaries, Managing
Expectations, and Challenging Unhelpful Guilt

Family is the heart of the Latinx culture. Within our family, we learn who we are, where we come from, and the legacies we are a part of. In the U.S., there is an emphasis on nuclear families whose goal is to raise children to become self-reliant and independent. However, for us Latinxs, our family relationships extend out much further past just immediate relatives. We rely on an extended network of people. Our goal isn't separation and independence. Our goal is interdependence. These extended support networks have been a major tool, allowing us to persevere despite difficult or challenging circumstances.

Many Latinxs grow up with one or both parents, and are also raised by grandparents, aunts, and uncles, and more. People tend to get the title *Tía* or *Tío* or *Primo*, even if technically in English their title would be more like great aunt, or second cousin. It's all family to us. Even trusted friends can become family through *compadrazgo*, godparenting. *Comadres* and *compadres* take responsibility for nurturing children, often with a focus on their spiritual education, and act as confidantes to the parents. *Compadrazgo* is another way of bringing even more families into the fold.

Each family member plays a part in our upbringing by

teaching us how to be a good person and decent member of our community. Each person will plant seeds they hope to develop as we grow. Family members often pray we will be successful, and that our success will allow us to contribute to the greater well-being of the entire family. We envision that our children can become teachers or doctors not just for their own gain or financial stability, but for how they can use that knowledge to support their family members. What is good for one will be good for all.

Like our ancestors, our families exist within cooperative and reciprocal support networks. Often families help each other with child rearing because we have a sense of loyalty, responsibility, and obligation. This structure can provide a loving and nurturing environment that supports a child's social and emotional learning and can be helpful to parents. Once we grow into adults, we will have learned the skills needed to engage in this cooperative system ourselves. These are skills like knowing how to both give and receive amiably; how to keep peaceful or balanced relationships with our family members, and how to fulfill our obligations. All things that come with being *bien educadx*, well brought-up.

Our development within our family system primes us to assume our role within our family. Each role comes with a purpose and a set of expectations. When everyone in the family fulfills their role, our family feels stable. Each family has their own definition of stability, and their own version of normal. Sometimes families become dysfunctional, and everyone plays a role in maintaining the dysfunction. Family can be one of our greatest resources, but when there is dysfunction in the family it creates an opening for emotional illness, spiritual hurt, and trauma.

Latinx people can value cooperative ways of family living and still have difficulty with the challenges that come from it. We may have experienced times when conflict, unfairness, or gossip was rampant within our family. Times when we have felt taken advantage of or overly burdened with familial obligations or responsibility. A challenge of this structure is that to achieve cooperation we must deprioritize independence in favor of interdependence. We must strike a balance between favoring the needs of the family, and our own personal needs and well-being—something that can become especially difficult when we are steeped in a dominant American culture that constantly tells us we should always prioritize ourselves first and defines success purely on an individual achievement basis.

Achieving healthy interdependence takes work, and it is not always easy to find the right balance. The balance between self and family can shift and change at different points in our lives. Other members of the family may not always understand or be supportive when the balance shifts towards prioritizing ourselves, even though this may be needed. Times this can become especially challenging are when we are going through life transitions that shift members' responsibilities, such as getting married, going to college, moving away, or having children.

Life transitions disrupt the equilibrium everyone is used to, and it can take time before a new balance is found. Flexibility is needed to maintain a healthy family and no person should ever have to continually sacrifice their own health or livelihood to meet others' expectations. When this occurs, we experience imbalance and role strain. Many Latinx people will experience role strain, especially when family expectations contradict our own personal goals or values or when caring for the family comes at the expense of caring for oneself.

Reflection and deconstruction

★ Who was involved in raising you? How did this shape your growing-up experience?

★ What are some of your family's strengths? What does your family do well?

★ Which of your current strengths or positive characteristics were nurtured by your family members?

★ What role(s) do you have within your family? What does it look like to play this role?

★ What is a story from your life that illustrates your role(s)?

★ What personal strengths have been developed because of your role(s)?

★ Have you ever experienced role strain like feeling limited or even harmed by the expectations that come with your family role? How have you managed role strain? What impact has it had on you? Does something need to change?

ENMESHMENT AND BOUNDARIES

Contrary to what many Western trained therapists believe, collectivist families are not inherently unhealthy, codependent, or enmeshed. Many families from cultures all around the world live and achieve healthy collectivism and interdependence. We find a sense of closeness that centers on warmth, time together, collective nurturance, and consistency. However, unhealthy dynamics can happen. Closeness that is more characterized by being controlling or possessive or closeness that happens because we're too anxious to be apart is not healthy. A sign of collectivism that has grown toxic is enmeshment.

Enmeshment happens when families get too close, and for the wrong reasons. Instead of the family being held together by strong bonds and relationships, members are held together by unhealthy attachments like negative emotions, trauma, addiction, or other shared problematic behaviors. If families only feel close when they are drinking together or gossiping together, they may be experiencing enmeshment. If everyone feels pressured to spend as much time together as possible despite never getting along, constant fighting, or being abusive to each other, this can be a sign of enmeshment. If family members are discouraged from having relationships outside the family, such as friendships with their peers, this can be a sign of enmeshment. In an enmeshed family, there is no room for individuality, and no acceptance of differences. We do not know where we end, and other family members begin due to lack of boundaries. This can lead to everyone sharing and participating in the same unhealthy behaviors.

Boundaries are necessary in any well-functioning family, even collectivist ones. Although some may think boundaries are the antithesis to living collectivism, healthy boundaries support healthy interdependence and prevent enmeshment. Boundaries lead to stronger relationships because they help prevent abuse or exploitation and allow us to maintain balance between ourselves and others. As Prentis Hemphill, embodiment educator, so beautifully stated, "Boundaries are the distance at which I can love you and me simultaneously."

Boundaries are the internal and external limits we use to understand who we are. Boundaries help us to know with whom we choose to share different parts of ourselves. Boundaries also help us to define roles and expectations in relationships. They dictate what we find acceptable in relationships, and when we feel safe. Some boundaries are flexible and situational or person dependent, while others may be more rigid or strict. There are several different types of boundaries, and we are constantly setting, negotiating, and renegotiating boundaries as our environments shift and our relationships change.

When families are enmeshed, individuals tend to lack boundaries and take on the emotions of others. When enmeshed family members complain to each other about others or gossip about others in the family, they spread their negative emotions. A conflict can quickly change from a problem between two people to a rift between several. A family member in a conflict may have unrealistic demands for support because it is hard for them to fathom that you could see a situation differently or feel differently than they do. They expect loyalty. Many of us have known of family members becoming estranged for fights that grew way out of proportion. Boundaries can become like a tourniquet and keep problems from spreading within the family and causing fractures.

Boundaries can also help prevent major splits between family members. Enmeshment often leads to resentment. When we cannot negotiate the right amount of giving and taking, or set healthy boundaries, we start to resent those around us. As that resentment festers, we start to see our family as the source of all our problems. If we don't have the tools to set boundaries and make changes, we may hide our anger or resentment as long as we can, but one day it becomes intolerable, and we shut ourselves off completely or leave. Alternatively, when we live with enmeshment, we may reject others when they try to set boundaries because we take it personally. Either way, the collective breaks down when we don't have enough space between members. Knowing and respecting boundaries can keep us from abandoning or being abandoned.

TYPES OF BOUNDARIES
Physical boundaries
This refers to personal space and physical touch. We have the right as individuals to decide how close others can get, who can touch us, and how. What is physically comfortable for one person may not be comfortable for another. All people have the right to their own physical boundaries, including children.

An example of respecting a physical boundary could be not forcing children to give everyone a hug or kiss when greeting them if they are not comfortable or do not want to.

Intellectual boundaries
This refers to thoughts and ideas. Healthy intellectual boundaries include respect for each person's thoughts or ideas without criticism or ridicule. It is okay to have different views, beliefs, or values from other family members.

An example of an intellectual boundary could be respecting and not criticizing a person's choice to use prescription medication to manage their mental health, even though you prefer holistic methods, or vice versa. Another could be respect for other people's personal interests and hobbies even if they don't align with your own.

Sexual boundaries

This refers to the emotional, intellectual, and physical aspects of sexuality. Healthy sexual boundaries involve explicit consent, mutual understanding, and respect between partners engaging in any sexual activity. Healthy sexual boundaries include respect for others' sexuality and sexual orientation. Sexual boundaries can also refer to limits regarding exposure to sexual material such as sexual jokes, innuendos, images, unwanted touch or advances, leering, or discussions. Children and minors are unable to consent to sex and should be protected from exposure to inappropriate sexual material or sexual behavior by adults. It is always the adult's responsibility to maintain appropriate and safe behavior with a minor, *no matter what.*

An example of a sexual boundary could be saying no to sexual activity you are not comfortable with. Respecting that boundary would mean your partner would not pressure or encourage you to engage in an activity you are not comfortable with or have said no to. Another could be refraining from making sexualized jokes or innuendos in the presence of children. Another example of healthy sexual boundaries includes teaching children the specific names of their body parts, and explaining who is allowed to touch these areas, for what specific reason, and who isn't. For example, a parent may be allowed to touch their genital area briefly as a part of a bath or to help clean them up after they use the restroom, but another adult cannot.

Emotional boundaries

These are the limits we set to protect ourselves emotionally. This can include who we share our personal feelings with and who we don't, or when we share personal or sensitive information with others and when we keep it private. Every person deserves privacy regarding intimate or sensitive information about their lives. Emotional boundaries include respect for others' feelings, even when they are different from our own. No one should be belittled or invalidated for how they feel. Emotions are subjective, and there is never a wrong way to feel. One person cannot dictate how someone else should or shouldn't feel.

An emotional boundary could be choosing not to share intimate details about yourself with someone you don't trust or don't know well. Respect for an emotional boundary could be finding someone's diary, and not reading it.

Time boundaries

This refers to how we choose to spend our time, including how much of it we give or share with others, how much time we need to maintain different responsibilities, such as work or family obligations, and how much time we need for ourselves. Healthy boundaries regarding time often mean finding an appropriate balance between everything listed above and understanding that that balance is different for different people.

An example of setting time boundaries could be a married couple deciding how much time they want to spend visiting family each week, and how much time they would like to spend at home together alone.

Material boundaries

This refers to how we share things like money or possessions, who we share them with and who we don't, how much we share, and when. Material boundaries can become a point of contention for many Latinx people who are expected to offer financial or material support to relatives. Material boundaries may need to be renegotiated at different points in our lives to maintain our own financial well-being while also meeting obligations to others.

A material boundary could be saying no to someone borrowing your car. Sticking to a budget can also be an example of setting material boundaries. Budgets create limits for spending or giving money to others and ensure personal needs are met first. Respect for a material boundary could be understanding how much money or financial help a person can give to you, without you pressuring them to give more.

MANAGING EXPECTATIONS

If you are the first person in your family to practice setting boundaries, know that some family members will disapprove. When we set boundaries, it does shift our relationships, and others will have their own perception about what you're doing. Unfortunately, sometimes people take it as a personal slight when boundaries are put into place. It can also take repetition for others to grow accustomed to boundaries so do not be disappointed when others need to be reminded—this is part of the process. If someone cannot respect your boundaries, even after being reminded, that may be a sign that you need a stronger boundary with them. Remember, the goal of boundary setting isn't to make everyone around you happy. It also isn't to tell others what to do. The purpose is to clearly define what you will or won't do or tolerate. It is to protect yourself from being hurt or taken advantage of.

✗ "Talk to me with some respect!" This isn't a boundary.

✓ "If you keep yelling, I am going to hangup the phone." This is a boundary because it is focused on what you will do in response to a behavior you can't accept.

✗ "Don't drink around me." This isn't a boundary.

✓ "I can't hang out with you if you've been drinking. If I think you have been, I am going to leave, and we can try again another day." This is a boundary because it is focused on what you will do in response to a behavior you can't accept.

✗ "Thanks for the invite to sleepover, not tonight, but maybe another time..." This is a vague response to a sleepover invitation, and leaves the door open to future invitations. If you are not comfortable with allowing your children to spend the night in certain places, it may be more helpful to communicate your boundary directly so there is no confusion later. Sometimes being passive is a response to feeling uncomfortable in the moment, but down the line this can make things harder.

✓ "Thank you for the invitation, but we don't allow our kids to spend the night anywhere without us. They can stay until bedtime." This is a boundary because it is focused on what you will do and are comfortable with.

Western psychology has historically painted collectivist cultures negatively by labeling us all as codependent and enmeshed simply due to our collectivist orientation. However, Latinx family culture is not inherently enmeshed or codependent. Western psychology ignores the healthy interdependence that our families are capable of and assumes that when people are reliant on each other it is automatically negative. We can heal enmeshment without replacing it with the toxic individualism promoted by Western culture.

We can achieve healthy interdependence when we allow for balance between the group and the person, can be flexible and understanding of others, and allow for differences between people. While navigating challenges or differences in the short term can be difficult, it serves the long-term goal of maintaining the family. Healthy interdependence is a protective buffer against some of the structural difficulties caused by an oppressive society and provides a safety net that isn't as readily available elsewhere in dominant U.S. culture.

Reflection and deconstruction

★ What are your boundaries? Take some time to reflect on each of the types of boundaries (physical, intellectual, sexual, emotional, time, and material), and figure out what those look like for you now.

★ How can boundaries help you to maintain safety? Remember that boundaries are not about what we want others to do, but what we will do to maintain our inner peace.

★ What are you scared you might lose if you set boundaries? What might you gain?

UNHELPFUL GUILT

Learning to grapple with guilt is a part of becoming an emotionally balanced Latinx person, and a useful skill for managing family expectations. We tend to feel guilty, a lot! Whether it is learned in our childhoods or piled onto us through religion, guilt is a feeling we need to learn to manage. Usually, guilt stems from feeling we should be doing more for others and less for ourselves. You haven't visited your grandmother as often as you think you should, guilt! You bought yourself a meal, but there is not enough to share with your siblings so guiltily you eat it alone in the car before going into the house. You get a new job and as you sit down in a comfortable chair you think of your mom working on her feet all day, guilt! Guilt is a normal part of our experience.

Guilt is even encouraged in collectivist cultures like ours, because it is an emotion that promotes accountability for wrongdoing and therefore supports group harmony. Helpful guilt is a feeling of discomfort when we have done something objectively wrong, violated a rule, or harmed someone. You might feel guilty if you steal money out of your grandfather's wallet or kick your dog after a tough day at work. Your actions were harmful and broke standards of moral behavior. This guilt can lead you to take accountability or change your behavior. This is helpful, and healthy.

Guilt can also be taken to an extreme and become unhelpful. Grappling with extreme guilt can easily become an emotional burden that no longer serves a purpose. If you feel responsible for things you have no control over or feel guilty when you have not done anything objectively wrong, you are experiencing unhelpful guilt. Many Latinx people I have worked with struggle with guilt, as they try to balance the expectations of two cultures.

Unhelpful guilt is feelings of intense discomfort about something we have done that either violates an unrealistically high standard, or when we take responsibility for something we did not have control over. When we are unable to resolve this guilt and find ourselves caught in a self-punishing guilty emotional cycle, we suffer with unhelpful guilt. Unhelpful guilt is often accompanied by self-blame, and harsh inner thoughts. If you feel guilty for resting, taking a day off, or for taking care of yourself, you are suffering from unhelpful guilt.

We typically learn unhelpful guilt during childhood. Because guilt is encouraged in collectivist cultures, our parents or caregivers may use it as a tool to control our behavior, even when they shouldn't. They may also struggle with unhelpful guilt themselves and pass it along to us. A child who comes home to find their depressed mother sobbing on the floor learns unhelpful guilt when she says, "I am crying because I do everything for you, and you don't even care. You are so ungrateful. I hate my life." The child takes on their mother's pain and feels responsible. This teaches the child that they are responsible for other people's emotions, even in indirect ways. This teaches the child that they are responsible for things they have no control over. This may teach the child to see themselves as bad. The child may clean the entire house trying to cure their mother's depression, which of course, they are unable to do no matter how spotless they get the house. Her sadness is more complex than one child's behavior. They are set up for failure and left with lasting, unhelpful guilt.

We may not be able to entirely free ourselves of guilt, but we can learn to recognize and manage unhelpful guilt to reduce its power over us. This can help us to separate what we can change from what we need to release and give ourselves a different perspective when unhelpful guilt tries to take over.

You can learn to challenge unhelpful guilt to reduce unnecessary suffering. When feeling guilty, do not immediately assume you have done something wrong, especially if you feel guilty regularly. Instead, ask yourself, "Where is this guilt coming from?" Once you have identified the source of the guilt, ask yourself, "Have I hurt someone or broken a law? Am I holding myself to an unreasonably high standard? Is this within my control?" If you find that you have directly hurt someone or broken a law, repair the hurt by apologizing, taking accountability, and changing behavior.

If you haven't harmed anyone, or are holding yourself to an unrealistic standard, this is unhelpful guilt. Practice talking to yourself kindly, like you would a loved one. Offer yourself comfort, and remind yourself that you are a human, and you can only be held accountable for what is within your control. Begin to practice releasing things that are outside your control. If this is difficult, check in with a friend, loved one, or therapist for support or another perspective.

REMINDERS FOR BALANCING FAMILY AND SELF

1. Be mindful of becoming a martyr within the family who always gives but never receives. Giving with no limits over time leads to anger, resentment, and depletion. It also feeds into the expectation that you will always be available, and never say no. Others will not consider your needs if you never do. Practice slowing down

before saying yes to helping others, and take the time to first assess if you have the time, money, or emotional space to meet their request. Consider if giving is taking away from your own well-being.

2. Remember also to ask for what you need, even if it is uncomfortable. We often think that others know what we need or how we feel, especially if we find ourselves anticipating the needs of others. However, this often sets us up for disappointment. No one knows how you feel or what you need unless you tell them. No one can read your mind. Asking for what you need gets easier over time and teaches you to engage in reciprocity. It will also show you who around you is truly participating in mutuality, versus who is only wanting to take. To be in healthy interdependence, you must prioritize your own wants, needs, and goals at times. It is important to be able to both give and receive to maintain the health of the family.

3. The responsibility for maintaining a family is never just one person's responsibility. It is a shared responsibility between everyone. Everyone benefits from having a healthy family, and every adult member should be invested in that goal and nurture those relationships. Each person's contribution may look different, and it will not be transactional or tit for tat, but it takes everyone to make it work for everyone.

4. Do not allow temporary discomfort to make you forget long-term goals. There may be times where we must do things others do not understand or like, but we know it is what is best in the long term. An example could be choosing to focus on school or a job training program instead of immediately going into the workforce. Our family may desire us to work as much as possible to financially contribute in the immediate moment, but we might understand that in the long term, school or job training will have more benefit to us and our family. This may require us to tolerate temporary discomfort

or tension for a long-term goal. Remember nothing lasts forever, and keeping a focus on the big picture can help us to not get bogged down by day-to-day conflicts. Ask yourself, "What makes more sense in the long run? How does my current sacrifice or discomfort get me closer to my long-term vision?"

5. Remember, it isn't your responsibility to end every unhealthy generational cycle that exists in your family. You can identify and practice unlearning dysfunctional patterns. You can make changes to your own beliefs, values, or behaviors. You can be more clear and compassionate in your communication. You cannot make others change who do not want to. When you make healthy changes, you plant seeds that will grow and bloom over many generations.

Reflection and deconstruction

★ Who do you consider family?

★ What is your experience when it comes to healthy collectivism, balance, and reciprocity? What works and what doesn't? What might need to change?

★ How does being with family or in community support your well-being? Is it worth it to you?

CHAPTER 10

FREEING OURSELVES FROM THE COLONIZATION OF GENDER

There can be no decolonization without depatriarchalization. In any decolonization process there is a constant practice of deconstructing, resisting, and transforming ways of life that are based on identity hierarchies. The patriarchal hierarchy is based on gender and is closely tied to sexuality. The default identity in this framework is to be a cisgender heterosexual male.[1] This is what we are all measured against. Deconstructing, resisting, and transforming strict gender roles, and the expectations and limitations that come with them, are liberatory acts of decolonization. And believe it or not, prior to colonialism gender didn't exist as we experience it today.

Gender refers to the social expectations associated with someone's sex. Today, our understanding of gender is dominated by the gender binary which states there are only two acceptable genders: male and female. Typical to many of the myths enacted by colonialism, the gender binary is said to

---

1   To be cisgender means your gender identity corresponds with the sex you were assigned at birth. For example, when you were born the doctor said, "It's a girl!", and today you continue to feel that you are a woman.

have a clear and scientific explanation. In this case, biological sex. However, the science of sex is much too complex to be reduced to two mutually exclusive categories.[2] In reality, gender is cultural and not biological. Every culture assigns certain behaviors, traits, or ways of being to people from different gender groups. What it means to be a man or a woman in one culture can look very different in another. In some societies, there are more than two accepted genders.

Gender identity comes from an internal sense we have that we are male, female, or another gender. As philosopher Judith Butler explains, "gender is an 'act,'" and it is one we must perform over and over. We act out our gender in how we dress, carry ourselves, and talk. *Machismo* and *marianismo* provide cultural scripts for these performances.

In our Latinx culture, *machismo* and *marianismo* are the dominant gender constructs that organize what men and women are supposed to be like. *Machismo* and *marianismo* are the products of multiple influences that have molded together since the beginning of colonization. *Machismo* and *marianismo* form Latinx gender role expectations, which in turn shape family role expectations, which then become individual members' attitudes, beliefs, and behaviors. Sometimes *machismo* and *marianismo* feel like the bars of a cage we have to struggle against.

Performing gender can make us anxious. When we perform well, we feel reassured or validated, and when we deviate from the script we are at risk of punishment. Society will regularly

---

2   Males usually have one X and one Y chromosome, and females usually have two X chromosomes, but there are many other possibilities. For example, some individuals have XXX (Trisomy X) or just X (Turner syndrome). Aside from chromosomes there are more than 25 genes that contribute to sex differentiation influencing the development of sex organs, the reproductive system, and how a body responds to sex hormones. For example, someone with androgen insensitivity syndrome (AIS) has XY chromosomes but is resistant to androgens, the sex hormones that influence the development of male organs. As a result, they can have female external genitalia and undescended testes, and no uterus. Sex and how someone experiences their gender identity is multifaceted and complex.

meet those who go outside the lines of the gender binary with violence. We see our *primo* getting spanked for playing with a doll or our *prima* being yelled at for not serving her father's plate, and we know to stick to the script. We learn the scripts whether we believe in them or not. Until enough of us consciously decide to make changes, *machismo* and *marianismo* will continue to influence our ideas about women, men, and people of all genders.

Reflection and deconstruction

★ What are some of the rules you've noticed regarding gender expectations that Latinos must follow? What about Latinas? What happens to Latinx people who don't follow these rules?

★ What are your beliefs regarding gender?

★ When did you first learn your gender? How did you learn it?

★ In what ways do you perform gender? What does it feel like in your body to be your gender? What does it mean to you to be that gender?

PRE-COLONIAL SOCIETIES AND GENDER

Pre-colonial societies were not organized around gender in the way we are accustomed to today. This can be a difficult idea to accept because gender has been presented to us and woven into our lived realities in such a way that gender can feel as natural as the sun and the moon. To imagine a world with different gender constructs requires us to stretch our imaginations to see a completely different world.

We must remember the Western colonial mindset is not timeless or universal. In *The Invention of Women: Making an African Sense of Western Gender Discourses*, Oyèrónkẹ́ Oyěwùmí writes that we cannot assume that gender as a social category based on biology was present in other cultures. The assumption that other cultures structured social categories around body differences is to impose a Western European mindset onto them. Other cultures have other ways of understanding themselves. Even if our ancestors thought of themselves as men or as women, those categories don't automatically have the same meaning or place in the social order. Oyěwùmí goes on to explain that gender was not an organizing principle for the Yoruba people of West Africa prior to colonization by the West. The primary principle of social organization was seniority, defined by relative age, not gender. Concepts of gender are not natural or biological. They are formed in a historical situation and are bound to culture.

Similarly, our Mesoamerican ancestors had their own notions regarding gender. They didn't share today's common view that women are subordinate to men. In *México Profundo: Reclaiming a Civilization*, Guillermo Bonfil Batalla describes the Mesoamerican society not as patriarchal, but as one where women were equal to men. Men and women's social roles were understood to be complementary. Life was organized around collective work, and women's contributions were equally valued. Each person in the group, regardless of gender, participated in collective decision making. Women were respected as the carriers of the culture who taught the group's ways of life to the children. In doing so, women ensured the continuation of their society, a highly respected contribution.

Our ancestors from the Andean region did not believe in a hierarchal relationship between men and women either. The idea of men and women's roles being complementary was grounded in their cosmovision. Bringing opposites into harmony without destroying either is seen as essential to all of existence. For example, the Earth's fertility was considered stronger when men and women worked together. In Quechua, this is referred to as *yanantin*, where male and female exist as complementary opposites like light and dark or inner and outer. They are opposite interdependent parts of a harmonious whole. In Aymara, the word *chachawarmi* (literally translates to man-woman) describes the nature of the cosmos and all of existence as male and female. All things are *chachawarmi* and have a counterpart. To have one part dominate or subjugate another destroys harmony and threatens all of existence.

Aside from gender roles, many Indigenous groups viewed femininity as sacred, and female deities as the creators of the universe. Paula Gunn Allen, in her book *The Sacred Hoop: Recovering the Feminine in American Indian Traditions*, says that the role of women in history has been minimized. She explains, "many American Indian tribes thought that the primary potency in the universe was female, and that understanding authorized all tribal activities, religious or social."

Sacred feminine energy was considered the source energy for all of creation, and as a result many Native American tribes used a matriarchal social organization. Paula Gunn Allen goes on to say that gender wasn't understood as primarily biological in Indigenous communities of Baja and the Southwest. In some groups, individuals' roles were determined by their temperament and interests, such as in the Mohaves and the Cocopah, who designated girls who chose boys' toys such as a bow and arrow to be male. The Yuma designated gender based on a person's dreams, and women who dreamt of war were designated and lived as men.

COLONIZING GENDER

So how did we get to where we are now? A patriarchal system where men have power, influence, and dominance over women. Women who are said to be naturally inferior. Like so many other things, it arrived with the colonizers. When the Spanish and Portuguese arrived, they brought with them a patriarchal gender system. They knew that one of the best ways to control a population was to create division and hierarchy. And so just like race, gender became another tool for social control and power guarding.

Relationships between men and women in the colonies were infused with a preoccupation with honor versus shame.

In *The Secret History of Gender: Women, Men, and Power in Late Colonial Mexico,* Steve Stern describes how the honor/shame codes set ideals for the outward expression of masculinity and femininity. The ideal man was a provider, protector, and authority. The ideal woman embodied obedience, acceptance, submissiveness, and moral sensitivity. While men were allowed to be sexually possessive, women were to remain virgins until marriage, then loyal to their husbands, and celibate if widowed. The gender codes of honor were supported by the church as tools of social control.

From the outset, non-white people could never attain the ideal womanhood or manhood taught in the colonies. A society based on their exploitation could never allow them to achieve the status necessary to be an ideal man or woman. Non-white men couldn't fulfill their roles as protectors, because they couldn't protect their families from the violence of the colonizers. Nor could they display authority over others, because of their place in the caste system. Non-white women were not seen as pure and saintly—quite the opposite. They were sexualized, forced to work in mines, fields, or as domestic slaves or servants, and were targets for abuse. Even so, during the colonial period and after, these influences took hold. Today, their legacy lives on in the current gender role expectations of *machismo* and *marianismo*.

MORE THAN MACHISMO

In the U.S., *machismo* and Latino masculinity are portrayed quite negatively. Stereotypes say Latinos are prone towards violence, bravado, hypersexuality, and alcoholism. Seared into our memories is when Donald Trump, announcing his first presidential run, said of Mexican migrants, "They are bringing drugs, and bringing crime, and they're rapists." They imagine *el borracho* from the *lotería* card wandering the streets inebriated and glistening with sweat, or perhaps they can't see past the Latinos they see in movies: *cholos* or drug traffickers. These stereotypes serve to further oppress and marginalize

Latinos as a scary other, and support racist rhetoric about Latinx people in the U.S.

In the American cultural lexicon, we rarely see the true representation of the men that many of us know, love, and respect. Men who are honorable, respectful, and loving. Men who take great pride in providing for their families, protecting them, and nurturing them. Men who gently teach their children the ways of the world while telling them stories and tending to the plants, the trees. Men who cry while the mariachi plays. *Cariñosos.* Men who are fully human. Latinos can of course express the negative aspects of *machismo*, to different degrees, but Latinos are so much more than a stereotype—when they are allowed to be.

Latino masculinity is an ancestral resource formed and reinforced long before the wounding of colonialism began. Latinx psychologists Hector Y. Adames and Nayeli Y. Chavez-Dueñas explain that the word *machismo* comes from the Nahautl word for *macho* "matti" which means "to be known." For the Mexica people, men proved themselves, or became known, by exhibiting virtues that were desired by their society—virtues like courage, vigor, fortitude, public achievement, discipline, and more, which are still important today.

In the book *Family Violence and Men of Color: Healing the Wounded Male Spirit*, author Jerry Tello looks to the Codices, recordings of Nahua culture by Fr. Bernardino de Sahagún, to understand Latinx ancestral masculinity. Tello explains that historically for a boy to become *un hombre noble* the family had to teach the values of the culture, build a strong moral foundation, and a sense of being rooted into these values. Tello explains that, based on the Codices and Indigenous elders' teachings, the true definition of being *macho* is to be dignified, a protector, nurturing, spiritual, faithful, respectful, friendly, caring, and sensitive.

These traits, expectations, and commitments live on today in Latinx culture, but there have also been changes, many of which come as a response to the wounds of colonialism. Under colonialism, many of the ways men were raised and achieved honor in their communities were taken away. Indigenous and African men were removed from their communities and forced to work in places like mines and plantations, resulting in a loss of culture, identity, and rootedness. Men were no longer able to protect their families. Women were brutally abused and exploited, many enduring physical and sexual violence, during the conquest and under colonialism, that produced deep shame. The fabric of the social order was ripped apart, resulting in not only community destruction, but also spiritual destruction.

Men suffered under the trauma of colonialism, and some absorbed the violence and indignation of the colonizers into their bodies and psyches. Stripped of their agency and authority, some internalized this violence where it seethed, turning into destructive anger. For some, this anger fueled a desire for justice and powered rebellions and uprisings against colonization. For others, this anger was numbed through alcohol or expelled onto the people they were taught to show dominance over—women and children. In doing so, men became both victims and perpetrators. This recycling of violence within the family lasted for generations as each hurt person sought to rid themselves of their pain by passing it on to others. Seeds of violent masculinity were planted and sewn over the coming generations, and violence within the family came to be normalized, or at least tolerated.

Today, we know that the traditional negative qualities of *machismo* like aggression and hypersexuality are harmful to men. Mental health research on *machismo* has found that Latinos who endorse dominance, sexism, and emotional restriction have higher rates of anxiety, are more hostile to others, and are less trusting. They tend to continue patterns of anger and domestic violence, perpetuating the intergenerational transmission of trauma.

Other studies have found that *machismo* is related to higher rates of depression, stress, and a lower likelihood of asking for help. *Machismo* can leave men sad, lonely, and unhealthy because it stops them from engaging in activities deemed too feminine, such as being vulnerable, expressing their emotions, or receiving support. When we can't find outlets for our pain and anger, we continue to turn it inward, becoming more angry, hopeless, and fatalistic.

It is important to say that the *machista* attitude is learned and can be unlearned, because it is socially constructed. We can, as a loving community, encourage all members, including men, to express themselves in a way that honors their families and ancestors, and reminds them that they too are sacred, complex, and deserving. We can recognize and process the underlying anger and frustration that stems from experiencing multiple oppressions so that these feelings aren't channeled into harmful behavior.

There are more adaptive ways to heal these soul wounds. We can return to our roots, and our rootedness, by creating spaces for men to come together, talk openly, and offer each other support and a path back to the true definition of *macho*. When surveyed, many Latinos agree that they would prefer a more fluid and flexible version of manhood—one that is less patriarchal, and less precarious; one that allows for a healthy expression of sacred masculinity, and a return to a more noble path.

Reflection and deconstruction

★ Think of a man in your life who you think shows healthy masculinity. This person might express emotions, be nurturing, be an active father, take on non-traditional roles or tasks, have sex lives that are based on consent and mutual enjoyment, or any other characteristic that you admire.

★ Why do you admire this person? What specific actions or behaviors of this person make you think they exhibit healthy masculinity? How do these actions or behaviors align with your own values and beliefs?

★ How can you challenge *machismo* in your own life? What

would it look like to free Latinos of these expectations? Would you treat yourself differently? Would you treat others differently?

★ Think of friends or family members with whom you could talk regarding *machismo* and masculinity in your community. Share your thoughts on what healthy masculinity means to you and the impact you think *machismo* has. Make sure to ask their thoughts and listen to their perspectives.

NI PUTAS, NI SANTAS—SÓLO MUJERES (NOT SLUTS NOR SAINTS—JUST WOMEN)

The cultural script for women, *marianismo*, was formed as the counterpart to machismo. *Marianismo* says the role of a woman is to be focused on her family and home life. Her energy should be used to be of service to her family. Many Latinas grow up serving their fathers and brothers, helping their mothers with household duties like cleaning, packing lunches, and watching children. It is obvious from a young age that they will have very different expectations placed on them than their brothers. While boys may be allowed to have lives outside the home, girls are often kept under their mother's watchful eye, and kept quite close. If she dares speak up or complain she might hear *calladita te ves más bonita,* you look prettier when you're quiet. Young Latinas are often taught that their self-worth comes from their ability to fulfill these expectations, and to remain pure. They are told that they could be easily ruined if the outside world gets to them.

Marianismo teaches women their purpose is to endure, and to sacrifice; to see their own happiness, pleasure, or fulfillment as something that comes after that of their husband and children, if it is to be even considered at all. When their husbands engage in infidelity or drink to excess, the responsibility shifts to the woman to keep her family together despite the misgivings of men. *Marianismo* transforms Latinas into martyrs. When women adhere to these expectations, their supposed reward is care and protection from the men in their family, and respect within their community—a reward that can come at a significant cost if it even comes at all.

The messages of *marianismo* are so ingrained that many of us have believed our mothers or grandmothers or sisters are this way because they like it. While the *mujeres* in our family may be invested in these role expectations as a route to self-worth in the community, we should never confuse that with making a free choice to live this way. Caring for one's family can be fulfilling, and being respected by your peers is a worthwhile goal, but power comes from the ability to choose. The penalties for failing to live up to these standards can be incredibly severe, and women who don't live up to *marianismo* risk rejection by their loved ones or community. Even if a person can perfectly embody this ideal, the abuse and suffering are built in. It's a gender trap.

ARCHETYPES FOR WOMANHOOD

When we think of how Latinas are expected to be in our culture, we can look at some of the *cuentos* or stories we are told growing up. Stories are a deeply powerful way of transmitting culture. These oral traditions teach us about three cultural archetypes for femininity: *La Malinche, La Virgen,* and *La Llorona.* Each have a part in the cultural narrative that explains to us what it means to be a woman. Each story transmits aspects of *marianismo* and ignores other factors that, if told, could become more empowering cultural narratives for Latinas.

La Malinche—The Traitor

La Malinche is a historical figure from the time of the conquest. She was an Indigenous woman mythologized as the ultimate traitor to her people. *La Malinche* was a translator and guide for Hernán Cortés. She could speak multiple languages and is said to have betrayed her people by assisting Cortés in defeating the Aztecs. She is blamed for bringing about the destruction of colonialism. *La Malinche* is described as the mother of the first *mestizos*, from her relationship with Cortés, making her one of our Latinx archetypal mother figures. The story of *La Malinche* teaches us to denigrate our Indigenous mother ancestors, and to associate Indigenous women with traitors and prostitutes. In Taino culture, Quispe Sisa, and in South America, the Andean woman, Anacaona, share similar narratives.

The often-untold story is that *La Malinche*, whose real name was Malintzin, was an enslaved child. She was born among Nahautl speakers, and then given to a Maya group after her father died and her mother remarried. She was taken by Hernán Cortés when she was 14. She was used for her language skills, and when Cortés was done using her, she was passed on to other men—a fate not uncommon to many Indigenous women of the time. She was a victim of one of the most brutal forms of violence used by the Europeans during colonization— rape. The story of Malintzin represents the shame of conquest that has been projected onto women. Many Latinas can relate to her plight—being judged for being a survivor, her victimization ignored, then being blamed for the horrific acts of men.

La Virgen—The Perfect Woman

Another trope that informs what Latinas are said to be is the Catholic figure *La Virgen*, mother of Jesus Christ. She was introduced by the Spanish as the Virgin Mary, and a symbol for womanhood. The most well-known apparition is *La Virgen de Guadalupe* who appeared to Juan Diego over four days in the year 1531. On this site today is the Basilica of Our Lady of Guadalupe, a Catholic church dedicated to the Virgin Mary, in Mexico City.

Not always mentioned in the story is that Juan Diego, also known as Cuauhtlatoatzin, was an Indigenous man who was a recent Catholic convert. *La Virgen* appeared where a shrine dedicated to the Mexica deity Tonantzin, Earth Mother, had formerly stood at the hill of Tepeyac. This was already an established site for pilgrimage, offerings, and festivals dedicated to Tonantzin. Different Indigenous peoples already traveled here to honor Tonantzin, and continued to do so even after the Spanish replaced her with the image of *La Virgen* we know of today, dressed in a cloak of the stars surrounded by sun rays, an image that carries both Christian and Indigenous symbolism. Many see *La Virgen de Guadalupe* as a blend of Aztec-Mexica goddess Tonantzin and the Virgin Mary.

La Virgen is a prominent figure throughout Latin America. In Colombia, she appeared as a Black Madonna and is named *La Virgen Morena de Monserrat*, in Paraguay she is known as the *Virgen de Caacupé*, and *Nuestra Señora de la Altagracia* in the Dominican Republic. *La Virgen de Los Angeles*, also known as *La Negrita*, is the patron saint of Costa Rica, while *Nuestra Señora de la Concepción Aparecida* is the patron saint of Brazil. These apparitions of a darker-skinned Mary wearing Indigenous symbols were critical in converting the Indigenous to Catholicism.

La Virgen is a complex figure. From the Catholic perspective, she is the ideal woman. She is everything Latinx culture tells women they should aspire to. She is simultaneously a virgin and a mother, creating an impossible standard for Latinas to live up to. *La Virgen* is associated with piety, submissiveness, and is viewed as docile and enduring. At the same time, *La Virgen* is also a cultural symbol of resilience, survival, and a connection to our Indigenous spiritual roots. She is our Earth Mother who has never left us. She embodies our historical veneration for sacred feminine energy. When we set aside the beliefs and values that have been forced onto us, we can restore women's place in society through her example.

La Llorona—The Suffering Woman

La Llorona is a prominent figure in Latinx oral history and storytelling. She is the archetype for the bad mother and suffering woman. She is said to have drowned her children in a fit of rage after learning her husband was cheating on her. She then took her own life. Her sad and lonely spirit now roams eternally as she cries into the night for her lost children. There are many variations to her story. In some versions, she is an Indigenous woman who had children with a Spaniard. When he refuses to marry her and leaves her for another, she kills the children and herself. In another tale, she is a migrant woman trying to cross the Rio Grande with her child. When the child accidentally drowns, she dies from the grief. Versions of this *cuento* are often told to us as children to instill fear so we won't wander off at night. We are told we can be taken away by *La Llorona* as a replacement for the children she lost.

La Llorona represents the concept of Latinas as long-suffering women who will endure endless pain. Stories of *La Llorona* are often tied to the extreme historical circumstances Latinas have had to survive, such as colonization or migration. Here she represents the collective pain of the people after colonization.

The story of *La Llorona* actually predates the arrival of the Europeans and colonialism. Similar stories are found in Aztec-Mexica mythology as well as in other cultures from around the world. Some have said that the story of *La Llorona* is one example of several prophecies that foretold the arrival of the Spaniards. *La Llorona* is said to be Cihuacoati, a motherhood and fertility goddess. She cried in fear of her children, the people, losing their spirit and destiny, which were seen as essential to maintaining balance and being well rooted. Indigenous practices of raising children focused on proper rooting where they were taught community values. *La Llorona*, to some, represents the collective losses of colonialism, including indigeneity and culture.

IMPACT OF *MARIANISMO*

Much like *machismo* harms men, *marianismo* harms women. Not only because these gender ideals can lead to structural oppression against women and increased violence towards women, but also because they lead to negative emotional well-being. *Marianismo* creates feelings of inadequacy and low self-worth as women struggle to measure up to impossible standards. *Marianista* attitudes are shown to lead to higher levels of depression, increased negative thinking, and negative emotions, resulting in a severe psychological burden. When women silence themselves to maintain family harmony, research shows that *marianista* behavior leads Latinas to have increased negative views of others, and feelings of cynicism and mistrust. Rejecting *marianismo* supports emotional well-being for women, healthier relationships, and respect for sacred femininity.

AGAINST THE STEREOTYPE

Another harmful aspect of *marianismo* is the narrowing of how Latinas are viewed. Latinas are flattened into one stereotype. The narrative of the passive, quiet, self-sacrificing woman dominates most other people's understanding of who Latinas are. The true history of Latinas as *mujeres poderosas* is suppressed. Latinas have never stopped engaging in the struggle for liberation and calling out for their rights and freedoms, despite the cultural and societal pressure to suffer quietly.

There exists a strong female revolutionary tradition and spirit in Latin America. Women fought colonialism, beginning with the conquest. During the final battles in Tenochtitlan, Indigenous women of Tlatelolco fought with the men against the Spanish. The women lined the rooftops carrying weapons and pouring water onto the Spanish soldiers. Later, in 1493, Natives destroyed the first Spanish community on Hispaniola, called La Navidad, in response to the Spanish invaders' sexual violence towards women.

During the slave trade, more slave ship mutinies took place on ships when there were many women on board. Once in the Americas, their rebellion continued. One rebellious woman was *La Virreina* Juana, who, after she escaped from slavery, founded Matudere, a community of escaped former slaves in today's Colombia. She ruled Matudere for almost 20 years. Warriors from Matudere carried out attacks on the Spanish and conspired with Africans living in the urban areas in acts of resistance.

Women fought to end colonialism as *guerrillas*, taking up arms in the wars for independence. Women like Cecilia Tupac Amaru, a direct descendant of Inka rulers, who led an Indigenous rebellion against the Spanish in 1780 or Juana Azurduy, a guerilla military leader who achieved the rank of lieutenant colonel in the fight for Bolivian and Argentine independence.

Later, when the newly established countries of the Americas and Caribbean went through periods of revolution, women were again engaged in the fight for increased rights, such as Elisa Acuña, a revolutionary who fought alongside Emiliano Zapata. Latinas have also fought against imperialism, and the destruction of their cultures and homelands. When the Zapatistas engaged in an armed uprising in 1994 against the Mexican government and neoliberalism, one-third of their army was comprised of women. Their declaration of war included the Women's Revolutionary Law, declaring rights and protections for women.

In all struggles that have existed in Latin America women have participated, and that legacy is carried forward today by Latinas who live in the U.S. There are women like Emma Tenayuca, a Mexican American labor organizer and civil rights activist who led a huge strike by pecan shellers in San Antonio, Texas, in 1938. And women like Sylvia Rivera, who led a riot in 1969 at Stonewall in New York City for queer rights, or Las Adelitas de Aztlán, who fought for Chicano rights and against the sexism of the Chicano movement in the 1970s. *Marianismo* cannot quell the revolutionary spirit of Latinas that drives our activism.

Reflection and deconstruction

★ Think of the important women in your life. Think of who they are, what they do, and what is expected of them. How much of this is influenced by *marianismo*?

★ What are your thoughts regarding the influence *marianismo* has on our culture?

★ Did you grow up with any of these *cuentos* about women? What did they teach you?

★ Think of women who have defied these stereotypes—perhaps women in your family, community, ancestral lineage, or others you know of (including yourself if you are a woman). What have these women done that you have admired? What rules did they break?

★ What does sacred femininity mean to you? How can we honor, nurture, and protect the sacred feminine?

QUEER AND TRANS LATINXS ARE SACRED[3]

One of the great losses associated with colonial patriarchy is the loss of reverence for queer and trans Latinx people. Historically, our ancestors understood that queer and trans people held a special place in society. They were viewed as the embodiment of the dualities that governed all of creation. They were understood to be reflections of the androgynous or gender fluid deities present in many of our ancestral religions. People like the *qariwarmi*, Andean third gender, who were shamans. *Qariwarmi* performed important rituals where they negotiated the tension between complementary opposites like the masculine and the feminine, the present and the past, and the living and the dead. They helped to preserve the gentle balance that prevented all of creation from being destroyed. Queer and trans Latinxs are sacred.

Our Mesoamerican ancestors knew gender was complex, and they didn't attribute a person's essential nature to the

---

3   I use queer and trans here in place of LGBTQ+ to describe any sexuality outside straight and any gender that isn't cisgender, and in recognition that terms like "gay" or "lesbian" are Western terms that serve to flatten or erase sexual orientation identities that exist in other cultural contexts. I use LGBTQ when that is the term used in source material.

body they were born into. Instead, they used *tonalli*, a person's day sign, to understand a person's inherent qualities. The day you were born was tied to your destiny, and your set of three companion animals. The body was understood to be unstable and affected by earthly and cosmological forces. Gender was not seen as fixed. It was tied to the labor one did, how one dressed, and how one spoke. One could change gender by changing clothing, hairstyle, speech, and taking on the labor of that gender. The basis of gender was not the body.

Like gender, we cannot assume that our current conceptions of sexuality are universal or timeless. In the book *The Flower and the Scorpion*, Pete Sigal explains that the concept of sexuality as a stable inner component of the self we have today didn't exist prior to the late 18th century. Now our current world is built to uphold the patriarchy that demands we be straight and cisgender. This system requires that people be reduced into clear categories, with neat labels. But the complexity of humanity doesn't bend well to such a reductionist system. Sexuality and gender are fluid and cannot be reduced to simple binaries like male/female or gay/straight. Every single person has their own unique expression of gender and sexuality regardless of the limits society attempts to impose.

While these categories may be made up, or socially created, they have real consequences. To exist as a queer or trans person today is to actively defy dominant norms regarding gender and sexuality. Because of this, queer and trans Latinx people are constantly given the message that their existence is wrong, both from dominant U.S. culture and Latinx culture. To be queer or trans and Latinx is to resist the implicit heterosexuality of *machismo* and *marianismo*. This can mean that queer and trans Latinx people face rejection, violence, stigma, and a denial of their right to exist.

Living under the additional marginalization that comes from being queer or trans creates an additional burden on the spirit. Queer and trans Latinx people may internalize feelings of shame, worthlessness, or inadequacy due to their treatment by society, or feel guilt for being unable to live up to the expectations others have of them—to be cis or straight. This burden weighs even more heavily when it must be carried without the support of one of our greatest resources: family, and community. The potential exclusion from a cherished social group isn't simply the threat of loneliness or loss of support, it is the threat of the death of a part of the self.

Cultural stigma contributes to the high suicide rate for queer and trans Latinx youth. According to the Trevor Project, Latinx transgender and non-binary young people reported significantly higher rates of suicide risk compared to cisgender Latinx LGBQ youth, with over half (53%) seriously considering suicide and more than one in five (21%) reporting a suicide attempt in the past year. Latinx LGBTQ young people have a 22% higher likelihood of a past-year suicide attempt compared to non-Latinx LGBTQ young people. These trends should not be perceived as a problem of suicidal individuals or mental illness, but as a social problem.

Suicidality of queer and trans Latinx people is a symptom of the breakdown of our society, and a breakdown of our connection to our ancestral heritages. It is a sign of the cultural amnesia that forced us to forget that we are all sacred, regardless of the categories we are forced into. Treatment of queer and trans Latinxs is a ripple of patriarchal colonial violence.

It is important for all people, and especially queer and trans Latinxs, to feel a strong sense of self and to be able to integrate their different identities. According to the research by the Trevor Project, LGBTQ youth who felt that their race or ethnicity was an important part of who they were had a 24% lower likelihood of a past year suicide attempt. Digressing from colonial ideas of gender and sexuality saves lives.

If a person feels they can be open with their family and continue to feel love and acceptance, their identity as a Latinx person and a queer or trans person will feel more integrated. If they face potential rejection, they may see these two parts of themselves as existing in separate realms.

For many of our families, there is often an avoidance of acknowledging sexuality at all, especially gay, lesbian, or bisexuality. Many Latinx people find themselves in a "don't ask, don't tell" situation with family members. For a queer or trans Latinx person to be less than a full family member is a violation of our ancestral legacy, and a sign of on-going colonization. We are allowing colonial categories of identity and colonial values to break up our families. This is a betrayal by the family of our queer loved ones, not the other way around.

To experience liberation, we must challenge ourselves to stop placing people into categories that define their worth and value as a person and control how they live. We must reject the idea that some human beings are more deserving or valuable than others. Although these concepts of gender and gender norms are deeply engrained, it would benefit us to remember that these strict constructs do not serve us, and they are not the ways of our ancestors. Liberating ourselves from the colonial mindset includes liberating ourselves from these strict roles, categorization, and gendered expectations.

As Latinx people seeking liberation, can we instead allow individuals to be more fully themselves without fear of rejection? Can we release the expectations of adhering to strict gender roles? Can we stop asking members of our family to sacrifice important and unique parts of themselves to satisfy these norms? Can we return to the ways of our ancestors where each person was encouraged to develop their own unique talents and capacities, knowing this will serve the advancement of the collective? I think we can.

Reflection and deconstruction

★ What messages about sexuality did you grow up with? What are your beliefs now?

★ What would it be like to be free of the expectations set by machismo and marianismo? Would you do anything differently? What would stay the same? How might those around you change?

★ Who in your family, community, or culture have you seen defy gender norms? In what ways? What was it like for them?

★ In a liberated future without systemic oppression will gender exist? Will we organize people by their bodies? Will we define people by their sexual orientation? How else might we define ourselves? How else could we structure families or communities?

CHAPTER 11

GETTING OUT OF SURVIVAL MODE AND BACK INTO THE BODY

LIVING IN SURVIVAL MODE

Healing from trauma is not a linear journey with a definitive endpoint. Our body, mind, spirit, and relationships will become like a garden that we will tend to through different seasons of healing. This journey will require us to come deeper into relationship with our own needs. Much like the earth's cycles shift and change, so will we. Taking good care of our interconnected cognitive, emotional, spiritual, physical, and relational needs is *the* healing practice.

Healing doesn't arrive in one drastic "Aha!" moment, but through small and repeated changes. Changes to how we think about ourselves, and our circumstances. Changes to the actions we choose to take, and changes in how we talk to and treat ourselves. To heal from trauma, we radically commit to our own worthiness, to our capacity to love and be loved, and to the value of our existence. We radically commit to the belief in our own ability to heal and transform ourselves and the world around us. We radically commit to each other and the interconnectedness of our healing and liberation. No one heals in isolation so we must fully commit to living as full a life as possible without limiting anyone else's.

Healing from trauma is a process and a practice that will

require consistent tending to over time. This doesn't mean one must suffer from debilitating flashbacks, uncontrolled anger, or excessive fear forever. It does mean that we acknowledge that living within traumatic and oppressive systems is something we will continue to contend with until we all achieve liberation. Engaging in a practice of self-nurture and community empowerment is part of our liberatory praxis. Although it isn't fair that we are tasked with healing ourselves and changing the world, *así es la vida*.

Remember that all trauma happens within the context of the different environments we live within. In previous chapters we've explored historical traumas like colonization, societal traumas such as systems of racism and patriarchy, community traumas such as institutional violence and stereotypes, and familial traumas like the strains of immigration and acculturation. The entry point to each of these types of traumas is the body. The body is the site where these forces interact and come forward to be expressed in the present moment. This is what it means to live with trauma. It means to experience traumatic stress reactions rooted in the past, but felt in the present moment, through your body. As Clarissa Pinkola Estés says in her book *Women Who Run with the Wolves*:

> The body remembers, the bones remember, the joints remember, even the little finger remembers. Memory is lodged in pictures and feelings in the cells themselves. Like a sponge filled with water, anywhere the flesh is pressed, wrung, even touched lightly, a memory may flow out in a stream.

When people think of trauma, they often think of either a war zone or a singular event where one is suddenly and unexpectedly in danger like a car accident, a housefire, or maybe a robbery. While these events can be traumatic, so can many other things we live through. Yes, trauma can include terrifying and dangerous events and circumstances, and it can also include experiences that are withheld from us, such as being nurtured, protected, validated, and cared for.

Reflection and deconstruction

Consider what events you have experienced that could be considered traumatic. You may have experienced these directly or been impacted if you witnessed or had a loved one have these experiences. Here are some common examples:

★ Domestic violence (verbal, physical, emotional, sexual, spiritual, financial)

★ Neglect as an infant or child

★ Verbal, sexual, physical, or emotional abuse as an infant or child

★ Parent arrested, incarcerated, or detained

★ Family member deported

★ Lack of nurturing as an infant or child

★ Not feeling loved or accepted by family

★ Lack of emotional safety in family

★ Lack of boundaries in family

★ Drug or alcohol use in the home during childhood

★ Extended separation from family or parents as an infant or child

★ Rejection by a parent

★ Being chronically discounted, humiliated, or shamed

★ Community violence

★ Institutional violence (e.g. child welfare system, school, police)

★ Physical assault (being slapped, kicked, hit, or beaten up)

★ Sexual assault or unwanted sexual experience

★ Witnessing another person being harmed or abused

★ Transportation accident (e.g. car, train, plane)

★ Robbery

★ Natural disaster (e.g. fire, flood, tornado)

★ Life-threatening illness or injury

★ Sudden or unexpected death of a loved one

★ Pregnancy (e.g. dangerous pregnancy or delivery, miscarriage, stillbirth, issues with fertility)

As you reflect on the different types of potentially traumatic experiences you've lived through you may notice that certain events continue to have an emotional charge as you think of them. You may find thinking of them brings an emotional intensity. You might notice your body being activated, such as feeling anxious, tense, or angry. You may also notice the opposite. Instead, you may feel a deactivation like a desire to shut down or withdraw, be numb, or just avoid thinking of the experience altogether. For other events from this list, you might notice that it feels quite different. You can remember your experience, but it feels like a regular memory. Sure, there may be a sense of sadness or regret that it happened, but it doesn't come alive in the same way or with the same intensity as the others. This is the difference between experiencing a traumatic event and living with trauma.

We go through many challenging or scary experiences in our lives, but the ones that keep us feeling stuck in survival mode, the events that come alive in our bodies through overwhelming emotion and sensation, are those that need more healing. Most likely when they occurred, we didn't have the support, the resources, or the safety to help us process what had happened and so we put it behind us. But these experi-- ences stay with us, and our body, mind, and spirit find it difficult to rest.

Remember, experiencing trauma does not mean there

is something wrong with you or that you are broken in any way. Trauma is unfortunately very common in our society. Although it may feel isolating or lonely, others have experienced the same things you have. Trauma makes us feel so lonely, but you are not alone in your experiences. Healing and recovery are possible.

Reflections and deconstruction

★ What does healing mean to you?

★ What would you like to see different or changed?

★ What would life outside survival mode be like?

★ To heal, what must be faced? What must be changed? What must be done?

★ What resources (personal, familial, cultural, ancestral, spiritual) will you draw from to find the courage and strength to carry you through the sacred journey of healing?

AUTOMATIC SURVIVAL RESPONSES: FIGHT, FLIGHT, AND FREEZE

Between stimulus and response, there is a space. In that space lies our freedom and our power to choose our response. In our response lies our growth and our happiness.

—AUTHOR UNKNOWN[1]

---

1 The quote is often attributed to Viktor Frankl, but it is from a book about Frankl's work called *Prisoners of Our Thoughts: Viktor Frankl's Principles for Discovering Meaning in Life and Work* (second edition) by Alex Pattakos, Ph.D. The author states they saw the quote in a book, but does not know the name of the book or its author.

Trauma leads to physical, emotional, behavioral, and cognitive responses that are designed to protect us from potential harm. These responses are called the fight, flight, and freeze stress responses. However, these responses are useful only in moments of true danger. When these reactions become consistent ways of being, they become problematic. We simply cannot live in survival mode all the time and have a full and pleasurable life. To heal trauma is to understand these responses and where they come from, and to create enough space within us that they are no longer able to hijack our mind and body when they aren't truly needed. To heal means to have choice in how we respond, and to free up energy to be used instead in service of our self and community actualization.

The body, mind, and nervous system work together to ensure our survival. These survival responses have been fine-tuned and passed down through our human evolution—they are not only strategies we learn from caregivers, community, and culture, but responses that are also inherited genetically. The fact that we exist today is due to the usefulness of these responses adapting and protecting our lineage over millions of years.

Our survival mechanisms function through our autonomic nervous system. Within the nervous system lies our personal internal surveillance system. Dr. Stephen Porges created the term *neuroception* to describe the way our nervous system scans our environment for signs of safety, danger, or life-threat without involving our conscious awareness. If our neuroception is picking up on signs of safety, we feel present, calm, capable, and can connect with those around us. If our neuroception picks up signs of danger, the alarm bell rings, sending signals throughout our body, and we automatically respond with fight, flight, or freeze.

Automatic stress responses are incredible tools for survival. But when we have experienced chronic lack of safety our nervous system has difficulty distinguishing between when we are safe and when we are in danger. This happens because we were in dangerous or invalidating conditions for so long or so often, we learned to live from a place of fight, flight, or freeze. It was never safe enough to turn the alarm off. Our nervous system stops paying attention to the signs of safety, and only focuses on danger. This is why we might find ourselves in situations where although we *know* we are safe, we still do not *feel* safe.

We might also stay in survival mode because we have too many traumatic experiences for our body and mind to make sense of. Our mind is unable to file away these experiences. Instead, they are kept in the forefront of our mind and are associated with danger. Details of the memory are encoded so that they become future warning signs that will set off alarms for our nervous system. After multiple traumatic events our nervous system associates too many stimuli with danger. Even when we are in a safe or secure setting, it does not take much to signal to our neuroception that danger *might* be present. Someone's tone of voice, the look on someone's face, a particular noise, a smell, or any other detail with similarity to a previous traumatic experience has the potential to trigger us, and we find ourselves back in survival mode. Our body reacts to false alarm after false alarm.

The reality is that many Latinx people live under chronic threat due to oppressive circumstances. Experiencing multiple oppressions makes us more vulnerable to social traumas like poverty or police violence, increasing the likelihood that we will experience multiple traumatic events, beginning at an early age. If you have a safe and nurturing home, family, or community that provides a respite from these experiences you have a buffer against the impact of these toxic stressors. This can help you to recover after these experiences, process them, and not carry them forward with you in such an intense way.

However, if growing up you did not have physical, emotional, or sexual safety, you were neglected, or you lived under chronic stress such as fearing a parent could be deported at any moment, the impacts of traumatic events may have influenced you even more deeply. You might not have had a safe respite to return to and recover. So now there may be difficulty perceiving accurately whether certain people or environments are safe or can be trusted. You may also have difficulty trusting yourself to make the right choice. The trauma attaches further into our self-concept, our ways of relating to others, and our ability to manage our emotions and control our responses.

MOBILIZING STRESS RESPONSES: FIGHT OR FLIGHT

Fight and flight are considered mobilizing stress responses. When the fight or flight stress responses are triggered, the body immediately activates, and uses increased energy to survive. Fight and flight are states of nervous system hyperarousal due to a perceived threat. Without thinking, our nervous system will command our body to either run from danger or fight back.

During fight or flight the brain releases stress hormones into the blood stream like cortisol and adrenaline. In fight or flight our blood pressure and heart rate increase, and more oxygen is pumped to our vital organs. Non-survival functions like digestion and immune system responses are slowed down to free up energy. Our thinking brain, the part that makes decisions, shuts down to allow the survival brain to take over. There is no time to weigh the pros and cons of fight or flight when true danger is present, and the body must react quickly.

When in fight or flight even our hearing changes. Our ears are more attuned to low-frequency sounds like a predator would make, and less attuned to higher frequency sounds like people's voices. This is often why it can be difficult to talk to someone who is in this state. They are not hearing you or processing your words in the same way as they would if they were in a calm or safe state.

Flight

The flight stress response is incredibly useful when we need to get away from danger. It is often the first response a healthy nervous system will choose in the face of true danger. Running away and putting distance between yourself and the danger can keep you safe from harm, whereas fighting carries risk of injuries. If you are a small kid getting bullied by a group of bigger, stronger kids, the flight response makes a lot of sense. The flight response involves running away from the threat or avoiding it altogether. It can help us escape from danger or reduce our exposure to stress. Some examples of the typical flight response are running away, hiding, or avoiding.

Living life in flight can look different. Being in constant flight mode can prevent us from resolving issues or facing our fears. An overactive flight response means typically using avoidance to cope, and unfortunately problems we avoid tend to fester and get worse. An overactive flight response holds us back from challenges, keeping us from experiences that help our growth. For example, flight can keep us from communicating when we have an issue with a loved one, due to our fear of what could happen. This robs us of developing necessary communication skills, and from an experience that could actually improve the relationship.

When flight becomes a way of being we may often feel anxious, panicky, worked-up, or shaky. We might have difficulty slowing down, focusing, and being present. In fact, it may be scary to do so. We tend to stay busy to avoid triggers or deeper introspection and reflection. Many people who tend to stay in flight mode feel a sense of impending doom that something bad will happen, and an impulse to always stay ready and vigilant. Flight mode can wreak havoc on the body, impacting sleep, digestion, and immunity, and resulting in us being more susceptible to illness, stomach problems, chronic pain, and fatigue.

Life in flight can take our thinking far away from the present moment and cause us to fall into unhealthy thinking styles. We look far into the future as we try to plan for every possible worst-case scenario. This thinking style is known as catastrophizing, and although it scares and worries us, we also feel as if it gives us a sense of control over what might happen. Not only do we focus on worst-case scenarios, but we also often disregard the potential for anything good to happen. This unhelpful thinking style is called discounting the positives. Because we try to be ready for anything, we can be hard on ourselves if we miss something or make a mistake, even when those things were outside our realm of control. We are often driven by perfectionism, which is an impossible standard to live up to and leads to beliefs of not being worthy or good enough. When we try this hard to always be in control, we are often left with the feeling that everything is out of control, a scary thought that retriggers us into flight mode.

Fight

The fight response is useful when we cannot get away and must face the danger head on. This response involves meeting the threat with aggression or resistance. The fight response can help us defend ourselves or protect others from harm, and the right amount of fight energy can help us to be assertive and take charge in a healthy way. Some examples of the fight response are yelling, arguing, hitting, and pushing.

Living life with an out-of-control fight response can cause many problems. We may often feel tense, on-guard, and defensive. Our anger, frustration, or rage are easily triggered, and we might take it out on others without thinking about the harm we're causing. Constantly having a guard up can be especially harmful in our close interpersonal relationships with friends and family. We may respond to things others consider small or unimportant with big emotional responses, often from a place of hostility or aggression, especially if we feel we have been wronged. We might magnify small things into big problems and have a hard time backing down from an unproductive argument. An out-of-control fight response can lead to violence and frequent conflict.

Our thoughts will focus only on winning or being right, making us unable to compromise. We will often blame others, often seeing the problem as something outside us, which prevents us from taking responsibility. Our inner voice can become highly critical of others, and towards ourselves as well.

Life with an overactive fight response means our emotional state is often shown as anger, even when underneath the anger we are sad, hurt, ashamed, or disappointed. This can make it hard to get our intimate and emotional needs met in relationships. Anger and aggression push people away when what we truly need is support, care, or for someone to see who we are beneath the shield anger creates. When others fear us, and feel they must walk on eggshells around us, they cannot develop the emotional connection or intimacy needed for closer relationships. We tend to want to dominate a situation or have power over others, because it makes us feel safer. Our unhealed trauma can be the mechanism through which we inflict trauma on others and keep ourselves from the healing power of relationships with others.

IMMOBILIZING STRESS RESPONSE: FREEZE

The freeze response is considered an immobilizing stress response, because the body shuts down to conserve energy and increase the likelihood of surviving a catastrophic injury. This is considered a hypoaroused state. Blood pressure and heart rate will slow, the body temperature will drop, and muscle tone will decrease. A person may appear limp or even lifeless. The brain will release endorphins that will help numb the body and increase the tolerance for pain. The thinking brain may shut off, and the person may seem faraway and unresponsive. This is a truly remarkable act by the body to preserve life as best as possible, and to take a person's consciousness away when they cannot physically leave.

Freeze

The freeze response is typically activated when escape or defense are not possible. To continue to struggle or resist could increase the likelihood or intensity of violence so to prevent increased harm our body shuts down and immobilizes. We may become still, quiet, lifeless, or zoned out. We may dissociate, disconnecting from the present moment in

Arousal zone	Response	Cognitive signs	Emotional signs	Physiological signs	Behavioral signs
High arousal: Mobilized	Fight	Focus on dominance, winning, or over-powering	Rage, anger, irritability, frustration	Increased heart rate, rapid breathing, muscle tension, sweating	Yelling, arguing, physical violence, defensiveness, intimidation
	Flight	Racing thoughts, ruminating, catastrophizing	Panic, fear, anxiety, worry	Increased heart rate, rapid breathing, sweating, trembling	Running away, avoiding, hiding, procrastinating
Low arousal: Immobilized	Freeze	Disorientation, confusion, amnesia	Numbness, dissociation, powerless, helpless	Decreased heart rate, shallow breathing, reduced movement, drop in blood pressure	Inability to move, feeling paralyzed, loss of speech

our mind, to be no longer fully present to experience what is happening. Some survivors describe a feeling of being outside their body, even watching from above. Others may have little or no recollection of a traumatic event due to the protection of dissociation. The freeze response is common for children who are often powerless during instances of abuse by adults, and during experiences of sexual assault.

Living life with an overactive freeze response can be incredibly difficult. This means operating from a consistent state of hypoarousal in the body. We may often feel tired and lethargic. Chronic low mood and depression can be indicative of life in the freeze response. We may have frequent episodes of dissociation, zoning out, or even losing time. We may gravitate towards activities we can use to dissociate, like endless scrolling, binge TV watching, a lot of reading, or excessive sleep. We may feel numb and disconnected from our bodies. We might isolate ourselves from loved ones, or even avoid relationships, due to fear of being harmed or of being a burden to others. Much of the fun and joy of life is difficult to connect to. Play, fun, and joy are states of excitement and arousal that can feel difficult to reach when in a chronic freeze response.

MY OWN STRESS RESPONSE SYSTEM

When we experience chronic or repeated traumatic events our stress response system can start to repeatedly use the same stress response system all or most of the time. Instead of using the most adaptive response for a given situation, we begin to over-rely on one or two. We may be fighting when it would be safer to run away, or we might find ourselves freezing over and over when it would be more useful to stand up for ourselves.

When we are stuck in one mode of being it feels as if it is just part of our personality. Someone who tends to use the fight response most of the time begins to be viewed by others as having an anger problem, while someone who is often in flight mode can come across as anxious or wound-up. A person often in freeze mode will struggle to be present and may seem withdrawn or depressed.

Reflection and deconstruction

★ Which of the automatic stress responses do you use more often? Do one or two of the automatic stress responses (fight, flight, freeze) tend to dominate or take over more often?

To manage our automatic responses, we must first understand not only what they look like, but what they feel like in our bodies. The more we know the felt sense of being in this mode, the more likely we are to catch it, creating space for us to nurture our nervous system and shift out of survival.

Complete these reflections for each response type (fight, flight, freeze), beginning with the most used and ending with the least used. It might be helpful to think of a time you were in this mode and take a few breaths to connect with the sense of it before answering. If it starts to feel overwhelming or too much, allow yourself to shift into your peaceful place. Return to your deep-breathing practice as often as you need.

★ *Relational:* What am I like when I am this response? How do I interact with others? How do others respond to me?

★ *Emotional:* What emotions are present?

★ *Cognitive:* What is my thinking like? What am I focused on? What do I tell myself?

★ *Physical:* What does it feel like in my body? What sensations do I notice? Where in my body do I feel these sensations?

★ *Triggers:* What types of things trigger this response in me? Remember that triggers can be certain experiences, sights, sounds, smells, or other reminders of past trauma. Sometimes the connection to a traumatic experience is clear, and sometimes it isn't.

Now that you have reflected on your automatic stress response system, take a moment to offer an expression of gratitude to your system. Although these responses may be causing you trouble now it is important to remember that these survival strategies exist because at one point it was the necessary response to ensure you survived a dangerous moment. This response exists because it once worked, and your nervous system desires nothing more than to keep you safe and alive. It could go something like this...

With one hand to heart and the other to your belly, take a few deep breaths: *I extend gratitude to myself, my body, and my mind, my fight/flight/freeze system for keeping me alive to experience this moment. Thank you for protecting me the only way you knew how. In this moment and going forward I choose to partner with you to live each moment more fully, and be more present in the now.*

SOOTHING THE NERVOUS SYSTEM

Now that we have a better understanding of our own automatic stress responses and what they feel like in our bodies, we can begin choosing practices to soothe the nervous system, turning down the alarms, and creating space for other ways of responding. Remember that these stress responses have been utilized repeatedly in your life, possibly within your family system, or for generations, so it will take time, practice, and frequent repetition for these changes to become embodied and accessible. This is the practice, the garden, the tending to over time.

The goal of these practices is to help the body to get back into a place of feeling more present and connected. This state is known as being within the Window of Tolerance (WOT), a concept created by Dr. Dan Siegel. The Window of Tolerance describes the optimal arousal zone for a person to function from in their daily living. When in their WOT, a person can think, feel, and make decisions.

As you can see in the graphic below when we are in fight

or flight our body is dealing with hyperarousal, and we will need to lower the level of stress energy in the body to get back into a more calm and present state, the WOT. Practices used here should make you feel like they calm or slow you down. Conversely, when we are in a state of freeze our body isn't experiencing enough arousal and we will need to bring energy and life back into the body to get up into the WOT. Practices here should make you feel like they energize you, reconnect you to feeling and sensation, and pick you up.

One thing to note is that the goal is not that we will always be in the WOT. We need our stress responses from time to time. The goal is that our nervous system will learn to respond more appropriately to what is happening around us. As we become more regulated triggers will move us out of the WOT less often or with decreased intensity. Even when we find ourselves mobilized or immobilized, we will have tools to gently guide our body back to where we want to be. The closer we can get to our WOT the more capacity we will have to be able to think about what is happening and process our emotions. This cannot happen unless we first learn to soothe our body, and work together with our nervous system.

Mobilizing responses: Fight or flight
Indicators: anger, rage, anxiety, tension, on guard, defensive, overwhelmed, panic, impulsive, racing thoughts. The body is experiencing too much arousal.

Window of Tolerance: Optimal arousal
Indicators: appropriately responsive, can think and feel, present, can connect with others, feel safe enough, engaged, can tolerate what is happening. The body is in its optimal state.

Immobilizing response: Freeze
Indicators: dissociated, disconnected, lethargic, fatigued, out of body, depressed, numb, slow processing, slow movements, zoned out. The body is experiencing too little arousal.

Figure 11.1: The Window of Tolerance

CREATING INTENTIONAL SAFETY WITH A PEACEFUL PLACE

We all need to experience safety. It is a basic human need, and a foundation for living a more fulfilled life. We may not have had a safe upbringing, or even have safe circumstances now, but we can intentionally create an experience of safety, peace, or calm for ourselves. The practice of creating a peaceful place nurtures our nervous system and helps tone down the trauma alarms that are over-ringing in our brains.

For this exercise, we can use to our benefit that fact that our human brains have a difficult time differentiating imagination from reality, especially when we imagine vividly. We can use this to our advantage to achieve our goal of spending more time outside survival mode. We can intentionally create a feeling of peace, calm, or security, allowing our nervous system to settle and practice being out of survival mode.

Imaginal exercise

Allow yourself to settle in somewhere comfortable, take a few deep breaths, and begin to imagine a peaceful place. It can be a place you've been before, seen on TV, or one you create with your imagination. It doesn't matter what type of place it is as long as it feels peaceful and secure.

Once you can visualize this place, start to notice every detail. Notice the colors, the sights, the sounds, the smells, the light, the temperature.

Imagine yourself fully immersed in this place, sensing how it feels on your skin as you walk around and take it all in.

If you need to make any additions or changes to make this place feel more peaceful or more secure, allow yourself to do this until it feels adequate.

Once the place is to your liking, spend a few breath cycles noticing what it feels like to be in a place that offers you full security and peace.

Spend as much time here as you need.

Remember that this place is a resource to you, and you

can return any time you need a moment of peace, calm, or security. Return to this place often and intentionally, allowing your nervous system to experience peace and calm more frequently. Consider this to be like strengthening a muscle, and over time your nervous system will be better calibrated to knowing the difference between times of peace and calm, and times of stress and danger.

Tip: If visualization in the mind's eye is challenging you can draw a peaceful place, create a virtual collage, use a picture, or find a YouTube video you like. Allow yourself to focus on the images, while making yourself aware of each sensation of being in this place.

Reflection and deconstruction

★ Have you ever felt safe? What is it like?

★ If you haven't experienced safety enough or often, what do you imagine safety would be like? Keep this in mind as you go through the next set of questions.

★ *Relational:* What am I like when I am safe? How do I interact with others when I feel safe? How do others respond to me?

★ *Emotional:* What emotions are present when I am safe?

★ *Cognitive:* What is my thinking like when I feel safe? Am I clear-headed, focused, or something else?

★ *Physical:* What does safety feel like in my body? What sensations do I notice?

★ *Resources:* What makes me feel safe? When do I feel safe? Who do I feel safe with? What brings me peace, comfort, or strength?

TOOLS FOR THE MOBILIZING RESPONSES

Deep belly breathing

Use the *respiración profunda* practice from the first chapter to settle your body and induce a sense of relaxation. Inhale for three seconds through the nose, pulling air deep into the belly towards your pelvis feeling the belly expand like a balloon. Exhale slowly out of the mouth for five seconds or longer.

Square breathing

A square has four sides. Picture tracing a square as you inhale for four seconds, hold your breath for four seconds, exhale for four seconds, hold your breath for four seconds. Repeat continuing around the square for four rounds (or more).

The mammalian dive reflex

Hold your breath and dunk your face into ice-cold water, making sure your nose, cheekbones, and eyebrows get wet. Hold for a few seconds to trigger the dive reflex which all mammals have. This decreases the heart rate, slows down breathing, lowers blood pressure, reduces anger, and relaxes the body.

Cold exposure

Cold temperature has been shown to soothe the flight/flight response.

- End your showers with a 30-second cold blast of water.
- Let pieces of ice melt in your hands as you breathe and watch them melt.
- Place an ice pack on the back of your neck or against your face.
- Let cold water run over your hands.

Tension and release

Practice tensing and then relaxing different parts of your body one at a time. You can start by squeezing your feet and curling your toes for a few seconds and then releasing, noticing any sensation of relaxation with the release. Move on to calves, then thighs, and glutes and continue moving up through different areas of the body until you've done shoulders and jaw, and scrunched your face. After a few moments of squeezing the muscle, release, and notice the sensation of relaxation. Once you've completed every separate body part, end with one full body tense squeeze before letting go into full relaxation.

The butterfly hug

Cross your arms and place your hands on your opposite biceps. Begin slowly tapping your hands on each arm, alternating left and then right, left and then right while taking deep breaths. It can help to play a free metronome at 60bpm from YouTube or Spotify to match the pace of the taps; 60bpm is a normal resting heart rate.

Calming sensory input

- Smell something with a relaxing scent, such as lavender.
- Listen to slow classical or instrumental music or steady drum sounds.
- Lie under a weighted blanket.
- Place a weighted stuffed animal or an 8lb bag of rice on your belly as you lie on your back.

Shake, move, or dance

Movement helps your body to discharge the extra stress energy of the aroused state. Because your body is already experiencing increased arousal, doing intense exercise or cardio could activate you further, so it is best to take a more gentle approach.

- Stand with both feet grounded and shake from the knees, either from side to side, or up and down with small bounces. Then take a turn shaking out each limb. Notice your breath and feel your body release tension and stress.
- Dance or sway to your favorite song.

- Practice yoga or tai chi to learn to pair breath to movement.
- Rock in a rocking chair or gently swing in a hammock.

TOOLS FOR IMMOBILIZATION: FREEZE
Five senses grounding exercise

Bring all your awareness back to the present moment through your senses. By taking stock of your surroundings, you can reorient yourself back into the present moment. Out loud if possible name five things you see around you. Then four things you can touch, and touch them. Next name three things you can hear. Take a deep breath, and name two things you can smell, and last, one thing you can taste. Repeat until you feel more connected or present.

Energized touch

Come back into the body by rubbing your hands together quickly for 10–15 seconds. Notice the energy and heat building between your palms. Next, distribute this energy around your body by sweeping your hands over your arms, down your legs, down your head and shoulders, as if you're dusting yourself off. Allow this energy to be cleansing. Let whatever can be released in that moment go. Imagine any negative energy, pain, or difficult emotion being taken from the body; allow the earth (or floor) to take it away from you. Notice what it feels like as you engage with your body, and shed what no longer serves. Thank *Madre Tierra* for taking this from you.

Connecting to your power

Try pushing firmly against the wall with your arms fully extended, your head up, and your right foot planted in front of your left. Use your energy to ground down through the feet. Notice the feeling of sturdiness in your body as you push. Push for five to ten seconds, then stop and notice your body. Switch feet so the left is forward and the right is back, and push again for five to ten seconds. If you are feeling strong emotions, focus on your breathing and the sensation within your body as you push against the wall. Feel your power.

Mindful walking

- Go on a walk and choose one favorite color to look for. As you walk, look out for anything this color and take a moment to notice its shape, texture, size, and other intricacies before continuing on. You can even take a picture of it.
- Take a mindful walk barefoot in the grass, noticing the sensations beneath your feet, on your skin, and between your toes. Notice the textures, temperatures, moisture, firmness, and any other sensations.

Activate the senses

- Eat something salty, spicy, tart, or sour.
- Listen to some upbeat music and move your body, shake your arms out, or stretch.
- Sing or hum to some of your favorite songs.
- Choose your favorite lotion or coconut oil and massage the soles of your feet. You can also use a massage ball or tennis ball to roll out on the sole of your foot.
- Use dry skin brushing towards the heart.

Warm up

- Warm up your body by wrapping yourself in a soft blanket.
- Put on warm and comfortable clothes and socks.
- Take a warm or hot shower.
- Make a hot herbal tea and notice how it feels as you hold it in your hands and take sips.
- Do some brisk movements or exercises like jumping jacks, high knees, or hold a plank for a few seconds if you are able.

Co-regulate

Our nervous system picks up on the state of those around us. Being near someone we feel safe and connected to can help gently bring us back into our WOT, whether we are feeling hyperaroused or hypoaroused. They may not be able to say or do anything to make us feel better, or fix our problem, but their presence can be a big help if we are open to it. Co-regulation is how we first learn how to regulate our emotions as infants. If a person isn't available, a pet can be a great substitute.

A REMINDER

Each of the above practices supports nervous system health and can help create increased capacity to manage stress and triggers. These practices can be used not only when we are triggered, but as a part of our regular practice of self-nurture. The more often you do something, the more likely you are to remember to do it when you are truly triggered.

Remember that these practices will take time and repetition to work. Choose a few you're interested in trying and practice them when you are feeling okay. Keep a log of the tools you've tried, and what they do for you. Keep the log somewhere you will see it often so that this stays fresh in your mind to practice.

When we are triggered it is very difficult to think and make decisions so we need to make these tools as accessible as possible. Many of the clients I work with put reminders of their tools on post-its around their room or keep their list as a phone lock screen or in a note. The less thinking we need to do when triggered the better.

Reflection and deconstruction

★ What practices will you try out? When? Scheduling self-nurture increases the likelihood we will do it. You can use a regular alarm on your phone to remind you to do some deep breathing a few times a day.

★ Are there things you already do that you find helpful?

★ How can you make these practices a part of your regular routine?

★ What are you willing to commit to doing to make changes and nurture your nervous system?

CHAPTER 12

LEARNING TO FEEL OUR FEELINGS, CHALLENGE NEGATIVE BELIEF SYSTEMS, AND PROCESS OUR TRAUMA

LEARNING HOW TO FEEL

The traumas we experience create disconnection in multiple places. Trauma fragments our memories splitting them into separate pictures, thoughts, emotions, beliefs, and sensations that flash without a sense of time or cohesion. As we practice nervous system regulation tools to take us out of survival mode, we develop greater capacity to be with our emotional experiences.

Learning to emotionally regulate means having awareness of our inner experience, feeling and naming our emotions, and learning to respond to our emotions and impulses in a way that honors the sanctity of ourselves and others. When we can be with these emotions without feeling consumed or dissociated, can support this emotional experience, and use curiosity to understand where our emotions come from, we become more regulated. Increased emotional regulation helps us to live more fully in the present and opens us up to new ways of engaging with the world we live in.

Emotional regulation is a liberatory skill. When our heart, mind, body, and emotions are connected and supported we spend less energy on managing suffering. We are more clear, focused, and communicative. When we understand how we feel we also come closer to understanding when our needs are being met, and when they aren't. We increase our capacity to challenge and make demands of the systems and institutions around us. We can be in community with others and engage in praxis because we can lean into our emotional regulation and communication skills when things get hard. We are less worn down by the personal, group, social, and historical traumas our people have endured, because we are clear eyed in our vision for transformational healing. We can taste liberation, and we want more of it, for everyone.

UNDERSTANDING EMOTIONS

One aspect of being a conscious being is to feel. These experiences of feeling are called emotions. How and when we experience an emotion is personal. Our personality, our history, and our culture all influence how we experience our feelings and how we show them. We were most likely encouraged or even rewarded for showing certain emotions, and restricted from showing others. We can never tell someone their feelings are wrong, and no one should ever tell us our feelings are wrong. Our emotions are based on our own complex subjective experience. Our emotions make sense when we have the tools to understand where they're coming from.

When we grow up in an emotionally unsafe environment our feelings can become something we try to fight, push away, or ignore. Often, we are given the message that our emotions are a problem. We are scolded for being angry, for feeling hurt, or for crying. We learn to hide, repress, and push away "problematic" emotions. We might even be forced to hide emotions some might see as positive, like pride, joy, or happiness, depending on the situations we find ourselves in. When these feelings have nowhere to go, they become trapped in our bodies, linger, and often emerge in negative ways, expressed through our behavior. We might take our feelings out on others by breaking rules or being defiant, or we might take them out on ourselves through self-harm or in the way we talk to ourselves in our mind.

One thing that few of us learn is that we can consider an emotion to be a flow of energy, much like an ocean wave. It will come into our body, building in intensity until it peaks, comes down, and completes the energy cycle just like the way a wave crashes on the shore and then melts back into oneness with the ocean. Emotions ebb and flow.

Our emotions linger because of how we respond to them, and our inability to process them. According to Dr. Jill Bolte Taylor, a Harvard trained neuroanatomist, the cycle of an emotion lasts 90 seconds unless something retriggers it. When we interrupt the emotional cycle by trying to push away the feeling, it persists. When we have a critical thought about the emotion, the way it feels in our body, or about ourselves for having it, the cycle begins again and then again.

Emotions need to complete their cycle to leave our body. In a perfect world, we wouldn't react to our emotions, and they would leave our bodies as quickly as they came; but we are complex humans, and this is most likely an unrealistic expectation. However, we can improve how we engage with our emotions and learn to gently release them instead of trapping them in our bodies. It starts with learning how to feel them in the first place.

How to feel your feelings

1. *Notice it:* Notice the sensations in your body with gentle curiosity. Use your awareness to locate where in the body the sensations are and describe them. Sensations can be described using things like size, texture, temperature, weight, and even color.
   - In this moment I feel a lump in my throat. It feels about the size of a golf ball.

- I am noticing heat rising in my face. My cheeks feel red hot. My hands and legs are shaky.
- My body feels heavy. It feels as if there is a black hole in my chest. I feel as if I'm sinking into it.

2. *Name it:* Based on what you're noticing, name the emotion or emotions that are present. If you are unsure, it is okay to guess. Naming the emotion reduces the intensity of the feeling and allows us to witness our feeling state without being consumed by it. This is one way to be with the emotion instead of identifying with it. Dr. Dan Siegel calls this practice "name it to tame it." Some tips:
   - Say "I feel..." and not "I am..." You feel this emotion and it is temporary. This emotion is not a permanent state of being.
   - An emotion is one word, such as "I feel *scared*" or "I feel *mad*" or bored or disgusted, and so on.
   - If you find yourself saying, "I feel as if...", most likely you are describing thoughts and not naming an emotion. For example, if you say, "I feel as if no one is listening to me," you are stating a thought. You can follow this up with "and because of that I feel..." to help yourself get to the feeling. For example, "I feel as if no one is listening to me, and because of that I feel lonely."
   - If you tend to use the words "good" or "bad" to name your feeling state, challenge yourself to be more specific. Both good and bad can mean too many things. The more specific the better. And remember, you can feel multiple feelings at once, even if those emotions seem to contradict each other.

   Some examples of naming feelings:
   - I feel as if no one is listening to me, and because of that I feel disrespected and lonely.
   - My body is telling me I feel afraid.
   - In this moment, I recognize that I am experiencing anxiety and fear.

- I feel sad.
- I am having thoughts that I can't handle this and I feel weak and helpless.
- I feel sad that I got broken up with, and at the same time I feel excited to spend more time with my friends.

3. *Accept it:* Gently put your hands on the place on your body where you notice the feelings most strongly, and practice accepting and allowing this emotion. You don't have to resist it, try to change it, or push it away. This may seem counterintuitive when you are struggling with a painful emotion, but acceptance clears the channel and allows the energy of the feeling to pass through to its peak and resolve.
   - In this moment, I practice acceptance. I can allow these feelings to be.
   - It is okay to feel how I am feeling right now.
   - I welcome these emotions as they come, and I gently release them as they go.

4. *Be with it:* Take a few breaths, maybe even visualizing the wave of emotion. Imagine the waves peaking and breaking onto the shore, completing their cycle. Allow yourself to gently ride this wave, using your breath as a guide.

5. *Release it:* As the emotion dissipates, consider anything you might need to support the feeling until it is ready to leave. You may need to move, breathe, cry, write, pray, light a candle, touch plants, walk, or use some of the self-nurturing tools you have practiced. You may also need support or connection from a friend or loved one. Remember that it is okay to ask for what you need. Sometimes we don't need or want a pep talk or advice— just someone's presence for a few minutes is enough.

THE ROLE OF NEGATIVE BELIEFS

Negative beliefs can be a big source of suffering. Trauma influences our beliefs about ourselves, others, and the world. When we experience traumas during our developing years or repetitively, these can become deeply held core beliefs, and eventually a lens we process our experiences through. Identifying negative core beliefs and seeing how they influence our lives is an important step to recovery, regulation, and healing.

The types of negative beliefs we have depend on the types of experiences we have, and how we made sense of them at the time. They tend to revolve around four realms: safety, responsibility, self-worth, and control. Typically, there is a root experience connected to a negative belief. That root experience caused us to strongly believe something about ourselves, and subsequent experiences reinforce it. We begin to operate as if that belief is true. We typically have more than one negative core belief. Later, current events that activate this belief become triggers. When we are reminded of this belief we feel all of the difficult thoughts, feelings, and sensations that come with it.

Below are some examples of common negative core beliefs. Notice that these are statements that refer to the core of who we are as a person. These are not thoughts or reflections on situations.

Safety	Responsibility/ Control	Self-worth	Belonging
I am never safe.	I am responsible for everything.	I am a bad person.	I am alone.
I can't be safe.	Everything is my fault.	I am not worthy.	I am invisible.
It's not safe to feel.	I am a failure.	I am defective.	I am not valued.
I cannot trust anyone.	I must be in control.	I am stupid.	I am different.
I cannot trust myself.	I am out of control.	I am not enough.	I don't belong.
I am helpless.	I am powerless.	I am too much.	I am not loveable.
I am trapped.	I have to be perfect.	I am unimportant.	

IDENTIFYING AND CHALLENGING YOUR OWN NEGATIVE BELIEFS

When reviewing the list above, you might have immediately noticed that certain beliefs had a strong emotional charge, or a sense of trueness for you. These are most likely your own negative core beliefs. However, if you're uncertain you can complete the exercise below to get a better understanding of what your core beliefs might be.

1. Return to your list of triggers from the "My own stress response system" section in the last chapter. Select one of your most common or powerful triggers.

2. As you think of the trigger, what negative belief(s) do you have about yourself *now*? What does this incident say about you *now*?

3. Put your answer into an "I am..." or an "I am not" statement, or select from the list above. You might have more than one negative belief for each trigger. This is very normal.

4. Instead of your negative core beliefs, what would you prefer to believe about yourself instead? What would be a more helpful belief? Remember to frame this in a positive way.

Here are some examples of shifting from negative to positive beliefs.

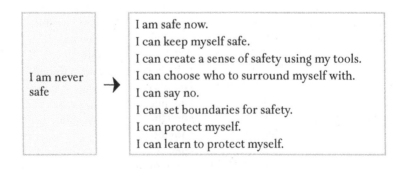

| I am never safe | → | I am safe now.
I can keep myself safe.
I can create a sense of safety using my tools.
I can choose who to surround myself with.
I can say no.
I can set boundaries for safety.
I can protect myself.
I can learn to protect myself. |

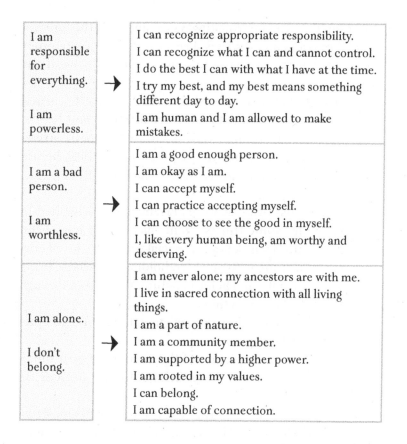

I am responsible for everything. I am powerless.	→	I can recognize appropriate responsibility. I can recognize what I can and cannot control. I do the best I can with what I have at the time. I try my best, and my best means something different day to day. I am human and I am allowed to make mistakes.
I am a bad person. I am worthless.	→	I am a good enough person. I am okay as I am. I can accept myself. I can practice accepting myself. I can choose to see the good in myself. I, like every human being, am worthy and deserving.
I am alone. I don't belong.	→	I am never alone; my ancestors are with me. I live in sacred connection with all living things. I am a part of nature. I am a community member. I am supported by a higher power. I am rooted in my values. I can belong. I am capable of connection.

POSITIVE BELIEF STRENGTHENING

Our positive beliefs do not feel less true because they are less true. They feel less true because our brain tends to focus on negative and traumatic events more so than positive and fulfilling ones. This is because our human brain has developed around survival and threat detection. Our brain is much less interested in keeping us feeling happy or joyful.

We must be intentional in developing and strengthening our positive beliefs. We must purposefully remind ourselves of our positive beliefs, and the experiences we've had that support them. Traumatic brain programming will minimize or ignore positive experiences, and this must be challenged. By intentionally focusing on our positive experiences, we create and strengthen the neuropathways in our brain that are not steeped in trauma and survival responses. We create other avenues for our brain to use to process and understand our experiences.

Positive belief strengthening is an exercise I learned through my Eye Movement and Desensitization and Reprocessing (EMDR) training, a treatment for traumatic stress. I often do this with clients in the preparation phase before doing any direct trauma processing. It goes like this...

1. Make a list of positive experiences you have had in your life. Some things clients have listed have been graduating from school, a special trip with a loved one, spending time with an elder, holding their baby, being in community, and being in nature. We then go through the events one at a time.
2. For this event, when you imagine it, what do you picture? Be descriptive.
3. As you hold the picture of the memory in your mind, what emotions and sensations do you notice? Be descriptive.
4. As you connect to this experience, what positive belief(s) feels true? Use the list above if you need ideas.
5. I then ask them to close their eyes, focus on the image, notice the positive emotions and sensations, and repeat the positive belief, while taking a few deep breaths.
6. To assist our brain in developing this memory, and creating a stronger connection to it, we use bilateral stimulation. From a seated position, place one hand palm down on each knee. Slowly and gently tap on your knees, right then left, right then left, as you engage in step 5. We call this "tapping it in" and it will help make this memory and the associated positive belief network even stronger. (You can also use the butterfly hug from the previous chapter or tap your feet right/left/right/left.)
7. Repeat with as many positive experiences as you like.

Return to this list often, add to it, and strengthen your brain's connection to positive or pleasant experiences.

FACING THE TRAUMA

Throughout this book, we have faced many things: the experiences of our ancestors and challenges within our families, and we've even explored the inner workings of our bodies and nervous systems. This has been difficult, yet necessary, work. What might feel even more difficult to face is your own trauma story. It can be very scary to name our experiences as trauma or abuse. The gravity of these words feels heavy. We may feel that using these labels turns us into a victim or makes us weak. Unfortunately, avoidance of our truth does not lead to healing. Avoidance makes things worse. Avoidance also leaves us fearful that if and when our truth is revealed, when someone brings up something that reminds us of our trauma, we won't be able to handle whatever comes next. The longer we avoid it, the scarier revisiting the past can feel, which means we are less likely to do the necessary healing work.

Some experiences must be faced. We need to process what we've experienced in a way that feels safe, affirming, and compassionate. Processing traumatic experiences helps us to make meaning of our experience, and to take something that is most likely a confusing mix of images, emotions, and sensations and turn it into a more cohesive narrative. We understand our lives through the stories we tell ourselves, and processing trauma helps us to take back control of our life's narrative.

There are many ways to process trauma: talking with loved ones, joining a support group, or in therapy using trauma-focused treatments like EMDR, Narrative Exposure Therapy, Internal Family Systems, or others. Processing trauma works when we can recall our experience in a place that feels safe, compassionate, and understanding. With this space, and the right support, we can start to alchemize the trauma. We take the fragments and pieces, and put them together, allowing us to feel, process, and understand the trauma. This process moves these experiences into the past where they belong.

Getting to the point of being able to talk to someone else or having therapy requires us to stop avoiding our trauma. One way to take steps towards healing and decreasing avoidance is through writing. These first steps can help us to grow more comfortable acknowledging our story and challenging narratives of shame, and open us up to other ways of seeing ourselves. This practice may clear just enough space that we can then go on to healing with a compassionate witness like a therapist or someone else we trust.

It is important to know that no one heals in isolation. While individual practices can help relieve the burden of trauma, the complete trauma-healing journey will always require connection with another. All human beings need to be seen, validated, affirmed, and cared for. We especially need to experience this in response to our painful stories. We can do the work and learn about healing, and develop our tools, but eventually we need to go back out into the world and see if what we've done holds up. We need to put our healing into practice in relationships with others and with community.

TESTIMONIOS

Testimonio is a method that began in Latin America in response to political oppression. *Testimonios* are a tool for finding our voice, documenting our experiences, and exposing injustice. By writing and sharing our stories, our testimony, we challenge the silence around trauma and the injustices we have faced, and the systems of oppression that make us more vulnerable to violence or abuse. The goal is to transform the trauma story from an account of shame or humiliation into one of dignity and truth. Writing your *testimonio* can help you to reclaim your life.

Prior to beginning the writing exercise, take some time to practice a moment of mindfulness. Take a few deep breaths to be present in the now and take note of what you are feeling.

If you find yourself experiencing a stress response, practice the tools you have learned so far. Remember that this practice will be difficult and will take time. Pause between each section to allow yourself to integrate what has come forward in your writing. Use your tools, and be kind and gentle with yourself.
To begin:

- Think of a traumatic experience you want to heal from and name the injustice that was done.
- When you are ready, begin with the factual details: what happened to you? Focus on the who, what, where, and when.
- *Once you are done, check in with yourself, and use your tools to manage any stress responses. Remind yourself you are safe and in control.*

Emotional exploration:

- What thoughts did you have during the event? What was going through your mind then? How did you make sense of what was happening then? What emotions did you feel during the event?
- *Once you're done, check in, and use your tools to manage any stress responses. Remind yourself you are safe and in control.*

Next, spend some time writing about how this experience has impacted you. You might consider how this experience shaped your beliefs about yourself or others, your sense of safety, trust, intimacy, or your relationship with your body.

- *Once you're done, check in, and use your tools to manage any stress responses. Remind yourself you are safe and in control.*

Reflection and deconstruction

★ Now, in present day and looking back, how do you understand what happened?

★ How did you survive this event? How did you cope with it?

★ When you think of the version of yourself that experienced this, how do you see them? How do you feel towards that version of your past self?

★ What do you know now that you didn't know then?

★ If a friend or loved one had gone through this instead, what would you say to them about it?

★ If you remember that this past version of you did the best they could at the time, and didn't know then what you know now, can you look at them with more loving eyes? Can you extend compassion?

★ What did that version of you need to know? Need to hear? Need to receive?

★ How can you honor those needs now?

The practice:

· Reading and re-reading what you have written, and then re-writing it will help you to process the experience, desensitize to the event—therefore reducing distress and trauma responses—and grow new insights. Remember to approach this exercise from a place of love and self-compassion, and to challenge any negative narrative you hold about yourself. This can be difficult to do alone, and when you are ready seek connection and spaces to share with others, to witness and be witnessed. Healing is possible.

ONE HEALING JOURNEY
Juan is someone who was deeply impacted by negative core beliefs formed from an early age. Juan was born in El Salvador. When he was four years old his mother left him with his grandparents to find work in the U.S. His family

didn't want to upset him so when she left they all told him she was going for a quick visit and would be back in a few days.

As time stretched on, Juan continued to ask about his mother, and was always told she would be back soon. Juan felt abandoned and thought constantly about where his mother could be and what she was doing. Juan decided he must have done something very bad for his mother to leave and not come back. He convinced himself that if he was good, she would come back to him. Juan helped his grandmother, said his prayers, and tried to remember to keep his hands and face clean like his mother had liked. But she didn't come back. Juan was convinced God was punishing him for how bad he must be, because only a bad little boy wouldn't have a mother. He didn't see her again until two years later when she sent for him. By then he believed very deeply that he was bad.

When they were reunited, Juan's mother tried to make up for lost time and bond with him but Juan was often moody and angry. He didn't like it when she hugged him, and he wiped away her kisses. He was terrified she would leave him again. He often stayed by the window and watched her walk to the bus stop to go to work, scared that would be the day she wouldn't come back. He anxiously watched the clock, and if she was even a few minutes late he became overwhelmed with fear. He couldn't trust her. He didn't think he could trust anyone.

Juan grew up, got an education and a good job at a school, but he struggled in his intimate relationships. When partners tried to get close to him, he would get irritable. He continued to think he was bad, so when people were nice to him, he was confused and distrusting. He didn't feel deserving of love, so their attempts at affection made him angry. Eventually he would blow up, and they would leave. This would confirm to him that he was bad, and that no one could be trusted. Over time, Juan grew tired of this cycle. He wanted to change it but felt powerless and unsure.

One day, Juan sat in on a presentation by the school's counseling department. They taught staff how to look for signs of trauma in their students. They talked about how many of the kids in his school were recent immigrants, and some had been separated from parents and family due to migration. They talked about how trauma impacts the brain. Suddenly things started to click for Juan, and he realized that he had experienced childhood trauma. Although his grandparents took good care of him, and his mother eventually sent for him, and provided him with a good life, he had still lived through a traumatic experience.

Juan decided to go to therapy. He found a local non-profit that offered trauma therapy and began meeting with a therapist. He learned about the connection between thoughts, feelings, and behaviors. His therapist helped him to identify the negative core belief of "I am bad" and "No one can be trusted." With this knowledge, he was better able to understand his triggers, and he learned tools to cope with his anger and his sadness. When he was ready, he wrote a *testimonio* about his experience as a young boy in El Salvador. With his therapist as a compassionate witness, he read and processed his writings. His therapist helped him to describe what it felt like to be a four-year-old without a mother. The therapist helped him to see why as a four-year-old he made sense of his situation in the way that he did, by blaming himself for her absence.

As Juan talked more openly about his thoughts and feelings and received support and validation from his therapist, he felt more compassion for his young self and his mother. He started to realize why that four-year-old believed his situation was a matter of good versus bad and he empathized with his younger self's lack of control. He began to research more about his home of El Salvador, and the lack of opportunity his mother had had there due to the country's instability. He realized she was forced into a difficult decision to be able to provide financially for him and his grandparents. He could finally understand his experience from a more mature perspective without reverting to the same beliefs he'd been using since childhood. He began to recognize more of his strengths, and the positive impact he had on young students. His depression and anger lessened as he moved through the world with greater capacity and more understanding.

CHAPTER 13

"HOY SEMILLAS— MAÑANA FLORES" (Today Seeds— Tomorrow Flowers)

Engaging *en la Lucha*, dreaming of *Buen Vivir*

Life in the U.S. can sweep you up into an ever-present state of urgency. Everything moves quickly, and we are taught to be results driven and solution focused, as if life happens on demand. The slower processes of healing and engaging in liberation work are the antithesis to this culture of urgency. This can be incredibly frustrating when we've been taught to rush. We want results now, we want to heal now, and we want change now. We want these to be tasks we can achieve all at once, rather than practices. But in the same way our healing from trauma comes in tending to the garden of our spirit daily through repeated acts, so will our liberation from the colonial mindset, soul wounding, and white supremacy culture.

Our liberation will come through praxis—continuous action and reflection, as we seek to change not only ourselves but also the world around us. We will plant many seeds, and patiently wait for them to grow into flowers. We have a collective responsibility to change the conditions of our society that lead to oppression and trauma. True healing, individual and community wellness, will come from the ending of social conditions that perpetuate harm. True healing will not come from the wellness industrial complex created by capitalism. We can't purchase our way into community wellness or liberation, no matter how many massages, gym memberships, self-help books, or meditation retreats we buy. True healing comes through liberation and co-creating a more equitable and just society, creating communities of care, and building networks of support.

Other ways of living are possible and can be realized. When we stay firmly rooted in our cultural values and embrace a decolonized mindset, we become powerful actors on our daily realities through the decisions we make, through our behaviors, and in our relationships. Our healing becomes plural, and ripples outward. As *Mujerista* theologian Ada María Isasi-Díaz explained in her book *En la Lucha/In the Struggle*:

> The way of life we embrace must lead to radical changes in the oppressive and exclusive practices in society. Our praxis must be, in the first place, firmly planted in the world of possibilities. Second, our liberation praxis is concrete. It refers to what happens in actual places, spaces, situations, and moments.

We can embody liberatory values in our ways of daily living. We can impact both the present and the future.

To engage in liberatory praxis we must be able to hold two complex notions simultaneously: the reality of the present and our hope for the future. In the present, we have *la lucha,* the concrete daily cultural and economic struggle of living as Latinx people; the daily existence of resistance to the dominant power system. And in the future, we have our greatest dream of something more—a future where we and all people have agency, support, and structures of society in place that promote wellness and equity instead of harm.

En la lucha, in our daily struggle, we focus on concrete liberatory acts. We live our daily lives with intention, and in our actions, and our interactions with others, we actively choose to prioritize our own value system and reject those that harm others. We purposefully uplift our culture, but never denigrate another's. We engage in solidarity with other oppressed peoples, and we do the hard work of finding paths of action to make change. *En la lucha* we foster and build community where we can engage in mutual support, and activism, and recognize that we are all connected. We build relationships, and create spaces that model the respect, reciprocity, and mutuality that we hope our future society will be built around. We dream and act our liberation into existence.

Reflection and deconstruction

★ Thinking of your daily life, in what ways do you engage *en la lucha*, the daily struggle against the dominant power structures of oppression? How does your daily existence defy colonialism, white supremacy, or the dominant power structures?

★ In your daily living, what seeds are you planting? What will they grow into?

BUEN VIVIR

We cannot achieve a liberated future if we do not challenge ourselves to imagine a society structured very differently from the society we exist within now. We need a radical vision for the future to inform our strategies for change and to guide our activism. Can we imagine a future where communities and societies are not structured around domination and hierarchy? One where social order isn't maintained through fear of punishment and harm via the state apparatus? One in which communities maintain standards of relationships built around respect and accountability? What will it look like?

In some places in Latin America, these conversations have begun to center around the concept of *buen vivir*, meaning the good life or good living. This philosophy comes from the organizing and activism of several Indigenous groups that are pushing for broad and sweeping social change. The concept is influenced by the Kichwa people of Northern Ecuador's concept of *sumak kawsay*. *Sumak* translates as harmony and plenitude while *kawsay* is life and coexistence. The Aymara people hold a similar notion, expressed as *suma qamaña*, meaning community in which basic needs are met and relationships, which even extend to the earth, are harmonious. *Teko porã* is a term in Guarani that means beautiful path or good living. Mayan Tsotsil and Tseltal peoples pursue *lekil kuxlejal*, a fair-dignified life. Philosophies associated with *buen vivir* are not exclusive to the Andes or Amazon and are based on cosmology and Indigenous ways of living in the present around the world, including *ubuntu* in Africa and *svadeshi*, *swaraj*, and *apargrama* in India.

In countries like Ecuador and Bolivia, *buen vivir* has been incorporated into the state constitution, allowing these concepts to have a greater influence on discourse and visions for the future. This led to the recognition of the rights of nature, the right to water, and banned privatization of water, as well as limited oil drilling in the Amazon.

Buen vivir emphasizes collective well-being over toxic individualism, and the importance of harmony between human beings and nature. *Buen vivir* recognizes the interconnectedness of all living beings, including humans, plants, animals, and the earth, and seeks to take us away from over-consumption and ecological exploitation. *Buen vivir* recognizes that the current economic system of endless growth and development promoted by capitalism is unsustainable on a planet with finite resources. *Buen vivir* asks us to imagine people who are whole and have their needs met living well together in community, and different communities living well together, while individuals and communities all live well with nature.

Buen vivir is influenced by several Indigenous philosophies and recognizes that there is no one true approach. Practices of good living exist throughout the world. *Buen vivir* imagines connecting different ways of achieving good living and bringing these ways into harmony. There is no rigid policy or institution of *buen vivir*. Communities throughout the world can imagine and structure their own ways of living well and harmoniously within their environments, and in communities that are non-hierarchical and are controlled by the community members. *Buen vivir* posits that we can move beyond exploitation of nature and accumulation of capital and instead structure society in ways that are designed to affirm quality of life, dignity, and solidarity. Alberto Acosta, an Ecuadorian economist, calls *buen vivir* "part of the long and complex emancipation process of humanity."

To achieve *buen vivir*, each group, people, community, and culture must develop and make explicit their most sacred values associated with good living. Rooted within these values will come the standards for forming relationships, and each relationship should seek to uphold these values. Our radical vision of *buen vivir* will guide us into being in safe, healthy, mutual, and respectful relationships with each other and our environments, and this will lead us into creating equitable social systems and conditions. Our people have long sought to realize this vision. In the writings of Subcomandante Marcos, a leader of the Zapatista movement, he reflected on the dream his community hoped to realize:

In our dreams we have seen another world, an honest world, a world decidedly more fair than the one in which we now live. We saw that in this world there was no need for armies; peace, justice and liberty were so common that no one talked about them as far-off concepts, but as things such as bread, birds, air, water, like book and voice. This is how the good things were named in this world. And in this world there was reason and goodwill in the government, and the leaders were clear-thinking people; they ruled by obeying. This world was not a dream from the past, it was not something that came to us from our ancestors. It came from ahead, from the next step we were going to take. And so we started to move forward to attain this dream, make it come and sit down at our tables, light our homes, grow in our cornfields, fill the hearts of our children, wipe our sweat, heal our history. And it was for all. This is what we want. Nothing more, nothing less.

Reflection and deconstruction

★ What is your radical vision for the future? What would a world without dominance and hierarchy be like? How does your vision align or not with the principles of *buen vivir*, such as community, harmony, and respect for nature?

★ What must you do in the short term to bring this about (one to five years)? What must you do in the long term (five to ten years)? What must you always do?

★ Who can you partner with in the creation of this vision? Who must you be in solidarity with?

★ What can you teach to others? What must you learn? Who can teach you?

PENDULATION BETWEEN REALITIES

Both *la lucha* and *buen vivir* deserve our consistent attention and prioritization. Sometimes this presents a challenge. It can feel difficult to find peace in a vision of the future when right now our people are being harassed by the police for street vending or are dying in migrant detention centers. Conversely, if we are too focused on the large-scale changes needed to accomplish *buen vivir* we may discount the importance of the small daily acts needed to slowly transform the system. We must hold both. Like our ancestors taught us, we must maintain our balance.

Here is an exercise I used to help my clients with this balance.

Put both hands out, palms up. Imagine in your right hand

you hold *la lucha*, the daily struggle of lived resistance. What are the qualities of *la lucha*? What does it ask of you? What does its energy feel like? As you describe it, close your right hand to a fist and hold it, taking a moment to connect with and feel the energy of *la lucha*.

Next, bring your attention to your left hand. Imagine in your left hand you hold *buen vivir*. What are the qualities of *buen vivir*? What does it ask of you? What does its energy feel like? As you describe it, close your left hand to a fist and hold it; really connect with the energy of *buen vivir*.

Now allow your attention to slowly go from your left fist to your right fist, spending a few breaths with each, and then back again. Notice what it is like to hold these two different practices at once. Notice what it feels like to be with one, and then with the other, pendulating back and forth between the different energies of the two.

This is the embodiment of daily practice of engaging in both. We are always holding both; even when we feel we might be focused on one, we are complex beings, and can hold many realities at once.

A FINAL *PALABRA*

In this book, we have explored many facets of the Latinx experience within the dominant Western and U.S. hegemony. I've tried to explain how, even with our incredible diversity, we have shared in some of the most transformative events that our modern world has ever gone through. We embody, as individuals, families, and communities, the complex nature of the current world system. We carry in our blood, our bones, our souls, the legacies of our ancestors—Indigenous, African, and European. The colonial project that has overtaken our world has intentionally disconnected us from ourselves— our history, our stories, our wisdom—and propelled us into traumatic experiences of oppression. What has allowed us to survive and even thrive despite it all has been our relationships and our culture. Our culture provides us with linkages to our ancestral wisdom, and has given us ways to experience love, joy, belonging, and healing in even the worst circumstances.

My intention with this book has been to shine a light on some of what has been lost or hidden, to help name the forces of white supremacy and colonialism that have influenced our ways of being and relating, in the hopes that by seeing them more clearly, we can free ourselves, our families, and our communities from their influence. My intention in writing this book is that if you have ever found yourself believing the lies you have been told about yourself, your people, and others who have experienced oppression that you can forgive yourself by seeing how complex and powerful the forces propagating these myths are. My radical hope is that this self-forgiveness frees us from any loyalty to the current system and incites us to use all our gifts, strengths, and resources to create something better. We have come very far, and we still have far to go, and we must go together.

La lucha sigue.

Appendix

The term Latinx isn't the first time we have had to navigate a potential shift in how our social group is defined. In 1977, President Richard Nixon's administration quite literally invented Hispanics. Prior to Directive No. 15, which defined new race and ethnic standards for federal statistics, there was no official term being used in the U.S. to categorize people who are now considered to be Hispanic, Latino, or Latinx. In fact, the term Hispanic was created to be an Americanized version of *hispano*, with the hope that its similarity to a Spanish word would increase acceptance.

Prior to becoming Hispanic, on the U.S. census we were counted as "White." We were quietly absorbed into the larger majority group and made invisible, at least from a numbers perspective. Regarding personal identity, most people at this time identified with the nationality of their family origin, such as being Salvadoran or Dominican. Suddenly, at least as a group, we were something new, different, and uniquely American. This category didn't exist anywhere outside the U.S.

In 1980, a mere 44 years ago, the federal government used the term "Hispanic" on the U.S. Census for the first time.[1] This addition was the result of decades of activism and lobbying by multiple groups led by the National Council of La Raza

---

1   The question on the 1980 census form was "Is this person of Spanish/Hispanic origin or descent?" The possible responses were: "No (not Spanish/Hispanic); Yes, Mexican, Mexican-Amer., Chicano; Yes, Puerto Rican; Yes, Cuban; Yes, other Spanish/Hispanic."

(NCLR), known today as UnidosUS. NCLR's goal was to secure funding for social programs in their communities, like job training. Without clear numbers on the population, it was difficult to prove that these communities were in need and at a socioeconomic disadvantage.[2]

The term Hispanic was met with pushback for several reasons. One of the key criticisms was that it defines a group of people by their ties to Spain, their former colonizer. It also leaves out people from Brazil, a South American country where Portuguese is spoken. As a result, in the year 2000 the term Latino was added to the U.S. census to now include anyone from Latin America regardless of language.

In the last two decades, the terms Hispanic and Latino have been used interchangeably to group together a large and incredibly diverse population of people living in the U.S. who are assumed to have related cultural origins. Neither term has ever been fully embraced by those it is meant to describe. A 2019 Pew Research Center survey found that only 39% used Latino or Hispanic to self-identify and instead preferred their family's country of origin to describe themselves. While we often see our identities as static, what we call ourselves and what others call us is constantly being renegotiated.

---

2   A Spanish language media network that later became Univision released a series of advertisements during the 1980 and 1990 census periods to teach people their new identity and encouraging these new "Hispanics" to fill out the census. The ads featured prominent "Hispanics" like Celia Cruz. Univision and Telemundo were instrumental in forming a broader consciousness for what it meant to be Hispanic and later Latino.

References

A Note on Language

Bishop, M. & Vargas, C. (2014, May 2). *The invention of Hispanics*. NPR. www.latinousa. org/2014/05/02/invention-hispanics.

Cohn, D. (2010, March 3). *Census history: Counting Hispanics*. Pew Research Center. www. pewresearch.org/social-trends/2010/03/03/census-history-counting-hispanics-2.

Engel, P. (2017). On naming ourselves, or: When I was a spic. *Cultural Dynamics, 29*(3), 193–201. https://doi.org/10.1177/0921374017727854.

Lopez, M. H. (2013, October 22). *Three-fourths of Hispanics say their community needs a leader*. Pew Research Center. www.pewresearch.org/hispanic/2013/10/22/three-fourths-of-hispanics-say-their-community-needs-a-leader.

Pelaez Lopez, A. (2018, September). *The X n Latinx is a wound, not a trend*. Color Bloq. www.colorbloq.org/article/the-x-in-latinx-is-a-wound-not-a-trend.

Ramos, P. (2020). *Finding Latinx: In Search of the Voices Redefining Latino Identity*. Vintage Books, a division of Penguin Random House LLC.

Salinas, C. & Lozano, A. (2021). History and Evolution of the Term Latinx. In E. G. Murillo, D. Delgado Bernal, S. Morales, *et al.* (eds), *Handbook of Latinos and Education* (second edition) (pp.249–263). Routledge.

Simón, Y. (2023, September 25). *Latino, Hispanic, Latinx, Chicano: The history behind the terms*. History. www.history.com/news/hispanic-latino-latinx-chicano-background.

Torres, L. (2018). Latinx? *Latino Studies, 16*(3), 283–285. https://doi.org/10.1057/s41276-018-0142-y.

Vidal-Ortiz, S. & Martínez, J. (2018). Latinx thoughts: Latinidad with an X. *Latino Studies, 16*(3), 384–395. https://doi.org/10.1057/s41276-018-0137-8.

Zong, J. (2022, October 26). *A mosaic, not a monolith: A profile of the U.S. Latino population, 2000–2020*. UCLA Latino Policy & Politics Institute. https://latino.ucla.edu/research/latino-population-2000-2020.

Introduction

Brave Heart, M. Y. H. (1998). The return to the sacred path: Healing the historical trauma and historical unresolved grief response among the Lakota through a psychoeducational group intervention. *Smith College Studies in Social Work, 68*(3), 288–305.

Brave Heart, M. Y. H. (2000). Wakiksuyapi: Carrying the historical trauma of the Lakota. *Tulane Studies in Social Welfare, 21–22*, 245–266.

Brave Heart, M. Y. H., Chase, J., Elkins, J., & Altschul, D. B. (2011). Historical trauma among Indigenous Peoples of the Americas: Concepts, research, and clinical considerations. *Journal of Psychoactive Drugs, 43*(4), 282–290. https://doi.org/10.1080/02791072.2011.628913.

Cerdeña, J. P., Rivera, L. M., & Spak, J. M. (2021). Intergenerational trauma in Latinxs: A scoping review. *Social Science & Medicine, 270*, 113662.

DeAngelis, T. (2019). The legacy of trauma. *Monitor on Psychology, 50*(2).

Freire, P. (2018). *Pedagogy of the Oppressed: 30th anniversary edition.* Bloomsbury Academic.

Gudsnuk, K. & Champagne, F. A. (2012). Epigenetic influence of stress and the social environment. *ILAR Journal, 53*(3–4), 279–288. https://doi.org/10.1093/ilar.53.3-4.279.

Lehrner, A. & Yehuda, R. (2018). Cultural trauma and epigenetic inheritance. *Development and Psychopathology, 30*(5), 1763–1777. https://doi.org/10.1017/S0954579418001153.

Menakem, R. (2017). *My Grandmother's Hands: Racialized Trauma and the Pathway to Mending Our Hearts and Bodies.* Central Recovery Press.

Ramirez III, M. (2004). Mestiza/o and Chicana/o Psychology: Theory, Research, and Application. In R. J. Velásquez, L. M. Arellano, & B. W. McNeill (eds), *The Handbook of Chicana/o Ppsychology and Mental Health.* Lawrence Erlbaum Associates Publishers. https://doi.org/10.4324/9781410610911.

Sharma, J., Shivers, C., & Bolinger, C. (2023, June). *A Cultural Framework for Generational Trauma.* American Counseling Association. www.counseling.org/publications/counseling-today-magazine/article-archive/article/legacy/a-cultural-framework-for-generational-trauma.

Sotero, M. (2006). A conceptual model of historical trauma: Implications for public health practice and research. *Journal of Health Disparities Research and Practice, 1*(1), 93–108.

Substance Abuse and Mental Health Services Administration (SAMHSA). (2014). *A Treatment Improvement Protocol: Improving Cultural Competence. TIP 59.* U.S. Department of Health and Human Services. www.ncbi.nlm.nih.gov/books/NBK248428/pdf/Bookshelf_NBK248428.pdf.

Volkan, V. D. (2001). Transgenerational transmissions and chosen traumas: An aspect of large-group identity. *Group Analysis, 34*, 79–97. https://doi.org/10.1177/05333160122077730.

Yehuda, R. & Bierer, L. M. (2009). The relevance of epigenetics to PTSD: Implications for the DSM-V. *Journal of Traumatic Stress, 22*(5), 427–434. https://doi.org/10.1002/jts.20448.

Yehuda, R., Daskalakis, N. P., Bierer, L. M., Bader, H. N., Klengel, T., Holsboer, F., *et al.* (2016). Holocaust exposure induced intergenerational effects on KFBP5 methylation. *Biological Psychiatry, 80*(5), 372–380. doi:10.1016/j.biopsych.2015.08.005.

Chapter 1: Grasping for the Roots: Civilizations Disrupted

Adames, H. Y. & Chavez-Dueñas, N. Y. (2017). *Cultural Foundations and Interventions in Latino/a Mental Health: History, Theory, and Within-Group Differences.* Routledge.

Anzaldua, G. (2012). *Borderlands/la Frontera: The New Mestiza* (fourth edition). Aunt Lute Books.

Bonfil Batalla, G. (1996). *Mexico Profundo: Reclaiming a Civilization.* University of Texas Press.

Chasteen, J. C. (2011). *Born in Blood & Fire: A Concise History of Latin America* (third edition). W. W. Norton.

Fery, G. (2020, October 23). *Burning the Maya books: The 1562 tragedy at Mani.* Popular Archeology. https://popular-archaeology.com/article/burning-the-maya-books-the-1562-tragedy-at-mani.

Fumudoh, Z. [@ziwe]. (2020, June 10). Throw every christopher columbus statue in the ocean and let that dizzy bitch think he discovered Atlantis [Post]. https://twitter.com/ziwe/status/1270742029065166849?lang=en.

Galeano, E. (1997). *Open veins of Latin America: Five centuries of the pillage of a continent* (C. Belfrage, Trans.; Twenty-fifth anniversary edition). Monthly Review Press.

Gordon, O. (2018, May 25). Andean cosmovision: The basics. Salka Wind Blog. https://salkawind.com/blog/archives/151.

Gordon, O. E. (2014). *The Andean Cosmovision: A Path for Exploring Profound Aspects of Ourselves, Nature, and the Cosmos.* Oakley E. Gordon.

Hudson, R. A. (ed.). (1992). *Peru: A country study.* GPO for the Library of Congress.

Hudson, R. A. (ed.). (1997). *Brazil: A country study.* GPO for the Library of Congress.

Hudson, R. A. & Hanratty, D. M. (eds). (1989). *Bolivia: A country study.* GPO for the Library of Congress.

Justeson, J. (2010). Numerical Cognition and the Development of "Zero" in Mesoamerica. In I. Morley & C. Renfrew (eds), *The Archaeology of Measurement: Comprehending Heaven, Earth and Time in Ancient Societies.* Cambridge University Press.

Kicza, J. E. (1993). *The Indian in Latin American History: Resistance, Resilience, and Acculturation.* Scholarly Resources.

Kilroy-Ewbank, L. (2017, September 12). *Mesoamerica, an introduction.* Smart History. https://smarthistory.org/mesoamerica-an-introduction.

Koch, A., Brierley, C., Maslin, M. M., & Lewis, S. L. (2019). Earth system impacts of the European arrival and great dying in the Americas after 1492. *Quaternary Science Reviews, 207,* 13–36. https://doi.org/10.1016/j.quascirev.2018.12.004.

Leon-Portilla, M. (1992). *The Broken Spears: The Aztec Account of the Conquest of Mexico.* Beacon Press.

Merrill, T. L. & Ramón, M. (eds). (1996). *Mexico: A country study.* GPO for the Library of Congress.

Mesoamerican civilization. (2023, September 15). Britannica. www.britannica.com/topic/Mesoamerican-civilization.

Molesky-Poz, J. (2006). *Contemporary Maya Spirituality: The Ancient Ways Are Not Lost.* University of Texas Press. https://doi.org/10.7560/713093.

Morgan, E. S. (2009, October). *Columbus' confusion about the New World.* Smithsonian Magazine. www.smithsonianmag.com/travel/columbus-confusion-about-the-new-world-140132422.

Murra, J. V. (2024, January 18). *Andean peoples.* Britannica. www.britannica.com/topic/Andean-peoples.

Suran, I. (2021, June 16). *The Andean cosmovision as a philosophical foundation of the rights of nature.* Notre Affaire à Tous. https://notreaffaireatous.org/en/the-andean-cosmovision-as-a-philosophical-foundation-of-the-rights-of-nature.

Chapter 2: The Hidden Truths of Colonialism

Brown, K. W. (2012). *A History of Mining in Latin America: From the Colonial Era to the Present.* University of New Mexico Press.

Burkholder, M. A. & Johnson, L. L. (2012). *Colonial Latin America* (eighth edition). Oxford University Press.

Chasteen, J. C. (2011). *Born in Blood & Fire: A Concise History of Latin America* (third edition). W. W. Norton.

Klein, H. S. & Vinson, B. (2007). *African Slavery in Latin America and the Caribbean* (second edition). Oxford University Press.

Parker, G. (1977). The Emergence of Modern Finance in Europe, 1500–1730. In C. M. Cipolla (ed.), *The Sixteenth and Seventeenth Centuries.* Harvester Press/Barnes & Noble by agreement with Fontana Books.

Rotimi, C. N., Tekola-Ayele, F., Baker, J. L., & Shriner, D. (2016). The African diaspora: History, adaptation and health. *Current Opinion in Genetics & Development, 41,* 77–84. https://doi.org/10.1016/j.gde.2016.08.005.

Stavig, W. (2000). Continuing the bleeding of these pueblos will shortly make them cadavers: The Potosi mita, cultural identity, and communal survival in colonial Peru. *The Americas, 56*(4), 529–562. https://doi.org/10.1017/S0003161500029837.

TePaske, J. J. & Brown, K. W. (2010). *A New World of Gold and Silver.* Brill.

Chapter 3: Creating Race in the Americas

Adames, H. Y. & Chavez-Dueñas, N. Y. (2017). *Cultural Foundations and Interventions in Latino/a Mental Health: History, Theory and Within Group Differences.* Routledge/ Taylor & Francis Group.

Aguilar, S. (2021, August 5). *Brown or white?: The dangerous disconnect between U.S. and Latin American media.* LatinaMedia.Co. https://latinamedia.co/brown-or-white.

Banks, T. L. (2006). Mestizaje and the Mexican Mestizo Self: No hay sangre Negra, so there is no Blackness. *Southern California Interdisciplinary Law Journal, 15*(2), 199–234, https://ssrn.com/abstract=790625.

Chasteen, J. C. (2010). *Americanos: Latin America's Struggle for Independence.* Oxford University Press.

Dalton, D. S. (2021). *Mestizo Modernity: Race, Technology, and the Body in Post-Revolutionary Mexico.* University of Florida Press.

Davis, D. J. (ed.). (2007). *Beyond Slavery: The Multilayered Legacy of Africans in Latin America and the Caribbean.* Rowman & Littlefield.

De Ferranti, D. M. (2004). *Inequality in Latin America: Breaking with history?* The World Bank.

Feliciano, C. (2016). Shades of race: How phenotype and observer characteristics shape racial classification. *American Behavioral Scientist, 60*(4), 390–419. https:// doi-org.csulb.idm.oclc.org/10.1177/0002764215613401.

Gates, H. L. Jr. (2011). *Black in Latin America* (first edition). New York University Press.

Harris, R. L. & Nef, J. (eds). (2008). *Capital, Power, and Inequality in Latin America and the Caribbean.* Rowman & Littlefield.

Hernández, T. K. (2022). *Racial Innocence: Unmasking Latino Anti-Black Bias and the Struggle for Equality.* Beacon Press.

Koehler, R. (2018). Hostile nations: Quantifying the destruction of the Sullivan-Clinton genocide of 1779. *American Indian Quarterly, 42*(4), 427–453. https://doi-org. csulb.idm.oclc.org/10.5250/amerindiquar.42.4.0427.

Manrique, L. (2016). Dreaming of a cosmic race: José Vasconcelos and the politics of race in Mexico, 1920s–1930s. *Cogent Arts & Humanities, 3*(1). https://doi.org/1 0.1080/23311983.2016.1218316.

Moraga, C. & Anzaldua, G. (eds). (1983). *This Bridge Called My Back: Writings by Radical Women of Colour* (second edition). Kitchen Table Press.

Morelos y Pavon, J. M. (1813). Sentimientos de la nación. In *Secretaria de Gobernación de Mexico.* www.bicentenarios.es/doc/img/8130914.pdf.

Noe-Bustamante, L. (2022, May 2). *Latinos experience discrimination from other Latinos about as much as from non-Latinos.* Pew Research Center. www.pewresearch.org/ short-reads/2022/05/02/latinos-experience-discrimination-from-other-latinos-about-as-much-as-from-non-latinos.

Ortiz, P. (2018). *African American and Latinx history of the United States.* Beacon Press.

Postero, N. G. & Zamosc, L. (eds). (2012). *Struggle for Indigenous Rights in Latin America.* Liverpool University Press. https://doi.org/10.2307/jj.3485509.

Reflective Democracy Campaign (2021). *White male minority rule by the numbers.* https://wholeads.us/work.

Telles, E. & Garcia, D. (2013). "Mestizaje" and public opinion in Latin America. *Latin American Research Review, 48*(3), 130–152. www.jstor.org/stable/43670097.

Twinam, A. (2015). *Purchasing Whiteness: Pardos, Mulattos, and the Quest for Social Mobility in the Spanish Indies.* Stanford University Press.

Vasconcelos, J. (1997). *The Cosmic Race: A Bilingual Edition.* United Kingdom: Johns Hopkins University Press.

Wade, P. (2010). *Race and Ethnicity in Latin America.* Pluto Press.

Chapter 4: Making the Invisible Visible: Unlearning White Supremacy Culture and Seeing Systems of Oppression

Baldwin, J. (1960). *They can't turn back.* History is A Weapon. www.historyisaweapon. com/defcon1/baldwincantturnback.html.

Bernardo, A. B. I., Levy, S. R., & Lytle, A. E. (2018). Culturally relevant meanings of the protestant work ethic and attitudes towards poor persons. *The Spanish Journal of Psychology, 21,* E40. https://doi.org/10.1017/sjp.2018.48.

Devos, T. & Banaji, M. R. (2005). American = White? *Journal of Personality and Social Psychology, 88*(3), 447–466. https://doi.org/10.1037/0022-3514.88.3.447.

Galdámez, M., Gomez, M., Perez, R., Renteria Salome, L., et al. (2023, April 20). *Centering Black Latinidad: A profile of the U.S. Afro-Latinx population and complex inequalities.* UCLA Latino Policy and Politics Institute. https://latino.ucla.edu/ research/centering-black-latinidad.

hooks, b. (2015). *Feminist Theory: From Margin to Center* (third edition). Routledge.

Izadi, E. (2019, August 6). *Honoring Toni Morrison through the words she shared with the world.* www.washingtonpost.com/arts-entertainment/2019/08/06/honoring-toni-morrison-through-words-she-shared-with-world.

Johnson, M. (2019). Oppression Privilege and Spiritual Practice workshop. Embodied Philosophy. www.embodiedphilosophy.com.

Katz, J. H. (1985). The sociopolitical nature of counseling. *The Counseling Psychologist, 13*(4), 615–624. https://doi.org/10.1177/0011000085134005.

Lucas, D. (2019). Measuring the cost of bailouts. *Annual Review of Financial Economics 11*(1), 85–108.

Mojica Rodríguez, P. D. (2021). *For Brown Girls with Sharp Edges and Tender Hearts: A Love Letter to Women of Color.* Seal Press.

National Museum of African American History and Culture. (n.d.). *Whiteness.* Smithsonian. https://nmaahc.si.edu/learn/talking-about-race/topics/whiteness.

Netherland, J. & Hansen, H. (2017). White opioids: Pharmaceutical race and the war on drugs that wasn't. *BioSocieties, 12*(2), 217–238. https://doi.org/10.1057/ biosoc.2015.46.

Okun, T. (2021). *White supremacy culture: Still here.* www.whitesupremacyculture.info/ characteristics.html.

Popuchet Quesada, K. (2020, September 9). *The violent history of Latin America is all about promoting whiteness (opinion).* Latino Rebels. www.latinorebels. com/2020/09/09/violenthistorylatinamerica.

Program on Intergroup Relations. (n.d.). *Social Identity Wheel.* University of Michigan. https://sites.lsa.umich.edu/inclusive-teaching/social-identity-wheel.

Sue, D. W. & Sue, D. (2016). *Counseling the Culturally Diverse: Theory and Practice* (seventh edition). John Wiley & Sons.

UnidosUS (2019). *Latinos and the Great Recession: 10 years of economic loss and recovery.* https://unidosus.org/wp-content/uploads/2021/07/unidosus_ latinosgreatression.pdf.

Young, I. M. (1990). Five Faces of Oppression. In I. M. Young (ed.), *Justice and the Politics of Difference* (pp.39–65). University Press.

Chapter 5: Soul Wounds

Alonso, P. (n.d.). *Autonomy revoked: The forced sterilization of women of color in 20th Century America.* https://twu.edu/media/documents/history-government/ Autonomy-Revoked--The-Forced-Sterilization-of-Women-of-Color-in-20th-Century-America.pdf.

Amiri, B. (2020, September 23). *Reproductive abuse is rampant in the immigration detention system.* American Civil Liberties Union. www.aclu.org/news/immigrants-rights/ reproductive-abuse-is-rampant-in-the-immigration-detention-system.

American Psychiatric Association. (2022). *Diagnostic and Statistical Manual of Mental Disorders* (fifth edition, text rev.). https://doi.org/10.1176/appi. books.9780890425787.

REFERENCES

Anzaldúa, G. E. (2015). *Light in the Dark/Luz en lo Oscuro: Rewriting Identity, Spirituality, Reality* (A. Keating, ed.). Duke University Press.

Balderrama, F. E. & Rodriguez, R. (2006). *Decade of Betrayal: Mexican Repatriation in the 1930s* (revised edition). University of New Mexico Press.

Blakemore, E. (2017, September 27). The long history of anti-Latino discrimination in America. History. www.history.com/news/the-brutal-history-of-anti-latino-discrimination-in-america.

Brave Heart, M. Y. H. (2000). Wakiksuyapi: Carrying the historical trauma of the Lakota. *Tulane Studies in Social Welfare, 21–22,* 245–266.

Brave Heart, M. Y. H., Chase, J., Elkins, J., & Altschul, D. B. (2011). Historical trauma among Indigenous peoples of the Americas: Concepts, research, and clinical considerations. *Journal of Psychoactive Drugs, 43*(4), 282–290. https://doi.org/10.1080/02791072.2011.628913.

Cacari Stone, L., Avila, M., & Duran, B. (2021). El nacimiento del pueblo mestizo: Critical discourse on historical trauma, community resilience and healing. *Health Education & Behavior, 48*(3), 265–275. https://doi.org/10.1177/10901981211010099.

Comas-Díaz, L. (2021). Afro-Latinxs: Decolonization, healing, and liberation. *Journal of Latinx Psychology, 9*(1), 65–75. https://doi.org/10.1037/lat0000164.

DeGruy, J. (2017). *Post Traumatic Slave Syndrome: America's Legacy of Enduring Injury and Healing* (Newly revised and updated edition). Joy DeGruy Publications Inc.

Duran, E. & Duran, B. (1995). *Native American Postcolonial Psychology.* State University of New York Press.

Duran, E., Firehammer, J., & Gonzalez, J. (2008). Liberation psychology as the path toward healing cultural soul wounds. *Journal of Counseling and Development, 86*(3), 288–295. https://doi.org/10.1002/j.1556-6678.2008.tb00511.x.

Estrada, A. L. (2009). Mexican Americans and historical trauma theory: A theoretical perspective. *Journal of Ethnicity in Substance Abuse, 8*(3), 330–340. https://doi.org/10.1080/15332640903110500.

Evans-Campbell, T. (2008). Historical trauma in American Indian/Native Alaska communities: A multilevel framework for exploring impacts on individuals, families, and communities. *Journal of Interpersonal Violence, 23*(3), 316–338. https://doi.org/10.1177/0886260507312290.

Lartey, J. (2018, July 5). *US immigration: What is ICE and why is it controversial?* The Guardian. www.theguardian.com/us-news/2018/jul/05/us-immigration-what-is-ice-and-why-is-it-controversial.

Linklater, R. (2021). *Decolonizing Trauma Work: Indigenous Stories and Strategies.* Fernwood Publishing.

Little, B. (2019, July 12). *The U.S. deported a million of its own citizens to Mexico during the Great Depression.* History. www.history.com/news/great-depression-repatriation-drives-mexico-deportation.

Martínez-Radl, F. B., Hinton, D. E., & Stangier, U. (2023). *Susto* as a cultural conceptualization of distress: Existing research and aspects to consider for future investigations. *Transcultural Psychiatry, 60*(4), 690–702. https://doi.org/10.1177/13634615231163986.

Magana-Salgado, J. (2014). *Detention, deportation, and devastation: The disproportionate effect of deportation on the Latino community.* Mexican American Legal Defense and Educational Fund. www.maldef.org/wp-content/uploads/2019/01/Deportation_Brief_MALDEF-NHLA-NDLON.pdf.

Montoya, M. (n.d.). *American Latino Theme Study: Law.* National Park Service. www.nps.gov/articles/latinothemestudylaw.htm.

Novak, N. L., Lira, N., O'Connor, K. E., Harlow, S. D., Kardia, S. L. R., & Stern, A. M. (2018). Disproportionate sterilization of Latinos under California's eugenic sterilization program, 1920–1945. *American Journal of Public Health (1971), 108*(5), 611–613. https://doi.org/10.2105/AJPH.2018.304369.

Sotero, M. (2006). A conceptual model of historical trauma: Implications for public health practice and research. *Journal of Health Disparities Research and Practice, 1*(1), 93–108.

Southern Border Communities Coalition (2023, February 10). *Border militarization.* www.southernborder.org/border_lens_border_militarization.

Whitbeck, L. B., Adams, G. W., Hoyt, D. R., & Chen, X. (2004). Conceptualizing and measuring historical trauma among American Indian people. *American Journal of Community Psychology, 33*(3–4), 119–130. https://doi.org/10.1023/B:AJCP.0000027000.77357.31.

Wills, M. (2019, March 26). The untold history of lynching in the American West. *JSTOR.* https://daily.jstor.org/the-untold-history-of-lynching-in-the-american-west.

Ybarra, M. (2022). Indigenous to where? Homelands and nation (pueblo) in Indigenous Latinx studies. *Latino Studies, 21*, 1–20. 10.1057/s41276-022-00389-w.

Chapter 6: *La Cultura Cura*: Grieving What Was Lost and Reclaiming What Remains

Acevedo, H. C., Shenhav, S., Yim, I. S., & Campos, B. (2020). Measurement of a Latino cultural value: The simpatía scale. *Cultural Diversity & Ethnic Minority Psychology, 26*(4), 419–425. https://doi.org/10.1037/cdp0000324.

Adames, H. Y. & Chavez-Dueñas, N. Y. (2017). *Cultural Foundations and Interventions in Latino/a Mental Health: History, Theory and Within Group Differences.* Routledge/Taylor & Francis Group.

Anzaldúa, G. E., Ortiz, S. J., Hernández-Avila, I., & Perez, D. (2003). Speaking across the divide. *Studies in American Indian Literatures, 15*(3/4), 7–22.

Arellano, J. E. (1997). La querencia: La raza bioregionalism. *New Mexico Historical Review, 72*(1), 31–37. https://digitalrepository.unm.edu/nmhr/vol72/iss1/6.

Burnett-Zeigler, I., Bohnert, K. M., & Ilgen, M. A. (2013). Ethnic identity, acculturation and the prevalence of lifetime psychiatric disorders among Black, Hispanic, and Asian adults. *U.S. Journal of Psychiatric Research, 47*(1), 56–63. https://doi.org/10.1016/j.jpsychires.2012.08.029.

Cervantes, J. M. (2010). Mestizo spirituality: Toward an integrated approach to psychotherapy for Latina/os. *Psychotherapy Theory, Research, Practice, Training, 47*(4), 527–539. https://doi.org/10.1037/a0022078.

Chasteen, J. C. (2011). *Born in Blood & Fire: A Concise History of Latin America* (third edition). W. W. Norton.

Côté, J. (2010). From Transculturation to Hybridization: Redefining Culture in the Americas. In A. Benessaieh (ed.), *Amériques Transculturelles/Transcultural Americas.* University of Ottawa Press.

Dunbar-Ortiz, R. (2014). *An Indigenous Peoples' History of the United States.* Beacon Press.

Esterman, N. (2020, April 10). *Embodied trauma conference 2020* [Video]. YouTube. www.youtube.com/watch?v=XVyCxUfnoXE.

Gordon, O. E. (2014). *The Andean Cosmovision: A Path for Exploring Profound Aspects of Ourselves, Nature, and the Cosmos.* Oakley Gordon.

Kananoja, K. (2018). Melancholy, Race and Slavery in the Early Modern Southern Atlantic World. In T. Laine-Frigren, J. Eilola, & M. Hokkanen (eds), *Encountering Crises of the Mind: Madness, Culture and Society, 1200s–1900s* (pp.88–112). Brill. https://doi.org/10.1163/9789004308534_005.

Klein, H. S. & Vinson, B. (2007). *African Slavery in Latin America and the Caribbean* (second edition). Oxford University Press.

Lakhani, N. (2022, June 20). *Honduras: Man who planned Berta Cáceres's murder jailed for 22 years.* The Guardian. www.theguardian.com/world/2022/jun/20/honduras-man-who-planned-berta-caceress-jailed-for-22-years.

Feliciano-Santos, S. (2021). *A Contested Caribbean Indigeneity: Language, Social Practice, and Identity within Puerto Rico Taíno Activism.* Rutgers University Press. https://doi.org/10.36019/9781978808218.

McNeill, B. (2015). The mestiza/o perspective. *Journal of Mestizo and Indigenous Voices, 1*(1), 1–7.

Mejías-Rentas, A. (2022, September 13). *The origins of 7 key Latin music genres*. History. www.history.com/news/origin-latin-music-styles.

Molesky-Poz, J. (2021). *Contemporary Maya Spirituality*. University of Texas Press. https://doi.org/10.7560/713093-006.

Murphy, J. M. (2012). "Chango 'ta veni'/Chango has come": Spiritual embodiment in the Afro-Cuban ceremony, Bembé. *Black Music Research Journal, 32*, 69–94.

Native Governance Center. (2022, April 15). *Blood quantum and sovereignty: A guide*. https://nativegov.org/resources/blood-quantum-and-sovereignty-a-guide.

Ortiz, F. A. (2020). Self-actualization in the Latino/Hispanic culture. *Journal of Humanistic Psychology, 60*(3), 418–435. https://doi.org/10.1177/0022167817741785.

Page, C., Woodland, E., & Levins Morales, A. (2023). *Healing Justice Lineages: Dreaming at the Crossroads of Liberation, Collective Care, and Safety*. North Atlantic Books.

Ramírez, M. (1983). *Psychology of the Americas: Mestizo Perspectives on Personality and Mental Health*. Pergamon Press.

Smith, T. B. & Silva, L. (2011). Ethnic identity and personal well-being of people of color: A meta-analysis. *Journal of Counseling Psychology, 58*(1), 42–60. https://doi.org/10.1037/a0021528.

Udo, E. M. (2020). The vitality of Yoruba culture in the Americas. *Ufahamu, 41*(2). https://doi.org/10.5070/F7412046833.

United Nations. (2007). *The United Nations' Declaration on the Rights of Indigenous Peoples*. www.un.org/development/desa/indigenouspeoples/wp-content/uploads/sites/19/2018/11/UNDRIP_E_web.pdf.

U.S. Government Accountability Office. (2022, December 15). *Women in the workforce: The gender pay gap is greater for certain racial and ethnic groups and varies by education level*. GAO. www.gao.gov/products/gao-23-106041.

Velasquez, R. J., Arellano, L. M., & McNeill, B. W. (eds). (2004). *The Handbook of Chicana/o Psychology and Mental Health*. Routledge.

Wills, C., Cuevas, C. A., & Sabina, C. (2022). The role of the victim-offender relationship on psychological distress among Latinx women: A betrayal trauma perspective. *Psychological Trauma: Theory, Research, Practice and Policy, 14*(1), 20–28. https://doi.org/10.1037/tra0000923.

Woodaman, R. (2017, December 28). *Bringing Taíno peoples back into history*. Smithsonian Magazine. www.smithsonianmag.com/smithsonian-institution/bringing-taino-peoples-back-history-180967637.

Worden, J. W. (2009). *Grief Counselling and Grief Therapy: A Handbook for the Mental Health Practitioner* (fourth edition). Routledge.

World Bank. (2023, April 6). *Indigenous peoples*. World Bank. www.bancomundial.org/es/topic/indigenouspeoples.

Ybarra, M. (2023). Indigenous to where? Homelands and nation (pueblo) in Indigenous Latinx studies. *Latino Studies, 21*(1), 22–41. https://doi.org/10.1057/s41276-022-00389-w.

Yoon, E., Chang, C. T., Kim, S., Clawson, A., *et al*. (2013). A meta-analysis of acculturation/enculturation and mental health. *Journal of Counseling Psychology, 60*(1), 15–30. https://doi.org/10.1037/a0030652.

Chapter 7: Immigration Stories Matter

Amann, E. & Baer, W. (2002). Neoliberalism and its consequences in Brazil. *Journal of Latin American Studies, 34*(4), 945–959. www.jstor.org/stable/3875728.

Beeton, D. (2022, April 12). *The Venezuela coup, 20 years later*. Center for Economic and Policy Research. www.cepr.net/the-venezuela-coup-20-years-later.

Borger, J. (2018, December 19). *Fleeing a hell the US helped create: Why Central Americans journey north*. The Guardian. www.theguardian.com/us-news/2018/dec/19/central-america-migrants-us-foreign-policy.

Castañeda, H. (2017). Migration is part of the human experience but is far from natural. *Nature Human Behaviour, 1*. 0147. https://doi.org/10.1038/s41562-017-0147.

Castañeda, H. (2019). *Migration and Health: Critical Perspectives.* Taylor & Francis Group. ProQuest Ebook Central. http://ebookcentral.proquest.com/lib/csulb/detail.action?docID=7040951.

Centre for Latin American and Caribbean Studies. (n.d.). *1992 reform of article 27 of Mexican constitution.* School of Advanced Study University of London. https://legalculturessubsoil.ilcs.sas.ac.uk/research-projects/legal-cultures-subsoil/1992-reform-article-27-mexican-constitution.

Central Intelligence Agency (2000, September 18). *CIA activities in Chile.* https://irp.fas.org/cia/product/chile/index.html.

Coatsworth, J. (2005, May 15). *United States interventions.* ReVista Harvard Review of Latin America. https://revista.drclas.harvard.edu/united-states-interventions.

Commission for Historical Clarification (1999). *Guatemala: Memory of Silence: Report of the Commission for Historical Clarifications.* Guatemalan Commission for Historical Clarification (CEH).

Farah, D. (1999). Papers show U.S. role in Guatemalan abuses: In declassified documents, diplomats describe massacres, CIA ties to army. *International Journal of Health Services, 29*(4), 897–899. www.jstor.org/stable/45131825.

Fernández-Kelly, P. & Massey, D. S. (2007). Borders for whom? The role of NAFTA in Mexico-U.S. migration. *The Annals of the American Academy of Political and Social Science, 610,* 98–118. www.jstor.org/stable/25097891.

Flores, A. (2017, September 18). *2015, Hispanic population in the United States statistical portrait.* Pew Research Center. www.pewresearch.org/hispanic/2017/09/18/2015-statistical-information-on-hispanics-in-united-states.

Gonzalez, J. (2011). *Harvest of Empire: A History of Latinos in America.* Penguin Press.

Janetsky, M. & Alemán, M. (2024, February 5). *"World's coolest dictator" Nayib Bukele claims El Salvador presidential reelection.* TIME. https://time.com/6660521/nayib-bukele-el-salvador-president-dictator-gangs-reelection.

Johnston, J. (2017, August 29). *How Pentagon officials may have encouraged a 2009 coup in Honduras.* The Intercept. https://theintercept.com/2017/08/29/honduras-coup-us-defense-departmetnt-center-hemispheric-defense-studies-chds.

Jordan, M. & Sullivan, K. (2003, March 22). *Trade brings riches, but not to Mexico's poor.* The Washington Post. www.washingtonpost.com/archive/politics/2003/03/22/trade-brings-riches-but-not-to-mexicos-poor/70d1823f-17d6-4587-b040-1b882c627ae2.

Krogstad, J. M., Passel, J., Moslimani, M., & Noe-Bustamante, N. (2023, September 22). *Key facts about U.S. Latinos for National Hispanic Heritage Month.* Pew Research Center. www.pewresearch.org/short-reads/2023/09/22/key-facts-about-us-latinos-for-national-hispanic-heritage-month.

McKinney, C. E. (2015). Twelve years a terror: U.S. impact in the 12-Year civil war in El Salvador. *International ResearchScape Journal, 2*(5). https://doi.org/10.25035/irj.02.01.05.

Menjívar, C. & Gómez Cervantes, A. (2018, August 29). *El Salvador: Civil war, natural disasters, and gang violence drive migration.* Migration Policy Institute. www.migrationpolicy.org/article/el-salvador-civil-war-natural-disasters-and-gang-violence-drive-migration.

Montoya, M. (n.d.). *American Latino theme study: Latinos and the law.* National Park Service. www.nps.gov/articles/latinothemestudylaw.htm.

Moslimani, M. & Noe-Bustamante, L. (2023, August 16). *Facts on Latinos in the U.S.* Pew Research Center's Hispanic Trends Project. www.pewresearch.org/hispanic/fact-sheet/latinos-in-the-us-fact-sheet.

Moslimani, M., Noe-Bustamante, L., & Shah, S. (2023, August 16). *Facts on Hispanics of Guatemalan origin in the United States, 2021.* Pew Research Center's Hispanic Trends Project. www.pewresearch.org/hispanic/fact-sheet/us-hispanics-facts-on-guatemalan-origin-latinos.

Moslimani, M., Noe-Bustamante, L., & Shah, S. (2023, August 16). *Facts on Hispanics of Salvadoran origin in the United States, 2021.* Pew Research Center's Hispanic

Trends Project. www.pewresearch.org/hispanic/fact-sheet/us-hispanics-facts-on-salvadoran-origin-latinos.

Office of Homeland Security Statistics. (2023, November 27). *Yearbook 2019: Table 39. Removed or returned: fiscal years 1892 to 2019.* U.S. Department of Homeland Security. www.dhs.gov/ohss/topics/immigration/yearbook/2019/table39.

Ormaechea, E. (2021). The failures of neoliberalism in Argentina. *Journal of Economic Issues, 55*(2), 318–324. https://doi.org/10.1080/00213624.2021.1907155.

Portes, A. (2006, July 31). *NAFTA and Mexican immigration.* Items. https://items.ssrc.org/border-battles/nafta-and-mexican-immigration.

Public Citizen (2019). *NAFTA's legacy for Mexico: Economic displacement, lower wages for most, increased migration.* Public Citizen. www.citizen.org/wp-content/uploads/NAFTA-Factsheet_Mexico-Legacy_Oct-2019.pdf.

Ribando Seelke, C. (2024, January 29). *El Salvador: Background and U.S. relations.* Congressional Research Service. https://crsreports.congress.gov/product/pdf/R/R47083.

Rugaber, C. & Associated Press. (2022, June 1). *U.S. job openings remain high, with nearly twice as many openings as unemployed people.* PBS NewsHour. www.pbs.org/newshour/economy/u-s-job-openings-remain-high-with-nearly-twice-as-many-openings-as-unemployed-people.

Sehnbruch, K. (2019, October 30). *How Pinochet's economic model led to the current crisis engulfing Chile.* The Guardian. www.theguardian.com/world/2019/oct/30/pinochet-economic-model-current-crisis-chile.

Shin, H., Leal, D. L., & Ellison, C. G. (2015). Sources of support for immigration restriction: Economics, politics, or anti-Latino bias? *Hispanic Journal of Behavioral Sciences, 37*(4), 459–481. https://doi-org.csulb.idm.oclc.org/10.1177/0739986315604424.

Tienda, M. & Sanchez, S. (2013). Latin American Immigration to the United States. *Daedalus, 142*(3), 48–64. https://doi.org/10.1162/DAED_a_00218.

United Nations Commission on the Truth for El Salvador. (1993). *From madness to hope: The 12-year war in El Salvador: Report of the Commission on the Truth for El Salvador.* www.usip.org/sites/default/files/file/ElSalvador-Report.pdf.

United States Agency for International Development. (n.d.). *Migration.* USAID. www.usaid.gov/guatemala/migration.

United States Census Bureau. (2020). *The Hispanic population in the United States: 2020 [Data set].* United States Census Bureau. www.census.gov/data/tables/2020/demo/hispanic-origin/2020-cps.html.

United States Select Committee on Intelligence. (1975). *Covert action in Chile 1963–1974.* Select Committee to Study Governmental Operations with Respect to Intelligence Activities. www.intelligence.senate.gov/sites/default/files/94chile.pdf.

Vasallo, M. (2002). Truth and reconciliation commissions: General considerations and a critical comparison of the commissions of Chile and El Salvador. *The University of Miami Inter-American Law Review, 33*(1), 153–182.

Vaughan, J. (2017). *Immigration multipliers: Trends in chain migration.* Center for Immigration Studies. https://cis.org/sites/default/files/2017-09/vaughan-chain-migration_1.pdf.

Waxman, O. (2018, November 30). *4 things to know about the history of NAFTA, as Trump takes another step toward replacing it.* TIME. https://time.com/5468175/nafta-history.

Weisbrot, M. (2015). *Failed: What the "Experts" Got Wrong about the Global Economy.* Oxford University Press.

Williamson, J. (1993). Democracy and the "Washington consensus." *World Development, 21*(8), 1329–1336. https://doi.org/10.1016/0305-750X(93)90046-C.

Williamson, J. (1990). What Washington means by policy reform. In *Latin American Adjustment: How Much Has Happened.* www.piie.com/commentary/speeches-papers/what-washington-means-policy-reform.

Wilson, M. (1993, November 23). *The North American Free Trade Agreement: Ronald Reagan's vision realized.* The Heritage Foundation. www.heritage.org/trade/report/the-north-american-free-trade-agreement-ronald-reagans-vision-realized.

Chapter 8: Twice as Perfect

Alba, R., Logan, J., Lutz, A., & Stults, B. (2002). Only English by the third generation? Loss and preservation of the mother tongue among the grandchildren of contemporary immigrants. *Demography, 39*(3), 467–484. https://doi.org/10.2307/3088327.

Alegría, M., Canino, G., Shrout, P. E., Woo, M., et al. (2008). Prevalence of mental illness in immigrant and non-immigrant U.S. Latino groups. *American Journal of Psychiatry,* 359–369. https://doi.org/10.1176/appi.ajp.2007.07040704.

Arce, J. (2022). *You Sound Like a White Girl: The Case for Rejecting Assimilation.* Flatiron Books.

Bacio, G. A., Mays, V. M., & Lau, A. S. (2013). Drinking initiation and problematic drinking among Latino adolescents: Explanations of the immigrant paradox. *Psychology of Addictive Behaviors, 27*(1), 14–22. https://doi.org/10.1037/a0029996.

Barajas, C. B., Rivera-González, A. C., Vargas Bustamante, A., Langellier, B. A., et al. (2024). Health care access and utilization and the Latino health paradox. *Medical Care.* https://doi.org/10.1097/MLR.0000000000002004.

Byers-Heinlein, K. & Lew-Williams, C. (2013). Bilingualism in the early years: What the science says. *LEARNing landscapes, 7*(1), 95–112.

Calzada, E. J. & Sales, A. (2019). Depression among Mexican-origin mothers: Exploring the immigrant paradox. *Cultural Diversity & Ethnic Minority Psychology, 25*(2), 288–298. https://doi.org/10.1037/cdp0000214.

Castañeda, S. F., Garcia, M. L., Lopez-Gurrola, M., Stoutenberg, M., et al. (2019). Alcohol use, acculturation and socioeconomic status among Hispanic/Latino men and women: The Hispanic Community Health Study/Study of Latinos. *PloS One, 14*(4), e0214906. https://doi.org/10.1371/journal.pone.0214906.

Dennis, J., Basáñez, T., & Farahmand, A. (2010). Intergenerational conflicts among Latinos in early adulthood: Separating values conflicts with parents from acculturation conflicts. *Hispanic Journal of Behavioral Sciences, 32*(1), 118–135. https://doi.org/10.1177/0739986309352986.

Franzini, L., Ribble, J. C., & Keddie, A. M. (2001). Understanding the Hispanic paradox. *Ethnicity & Disease, 11*(3), 496–518.

Geiger, G., Kiel, L., Horiguchi, M., Martinez-Aceves, C., et al. (2024). Latinas in medicine: Evaluating and understanding the experience of Latinas in medical education: A cross sectional survey. *BMC Medical Education, 24*(1), 4. https://doi.org/10.1186/s12909-023-04982-y.

Heilemann, M. V., Lee, K. A., & Kury, F. S. (2002). Strengths and vulnerabilities of women of Mexican descent in relation to depressive symptoms. *Nursing Research, 51*(3), 175–182. https://doi.org/10.1097/00006199-200205000-00006.

Liu, W. M., Liu, R. Z., Garrison, Y. L., Kim, J. Y. C., et al. (2019). Racial trauma, microaggressions, and becoming racially innocuous: The role of acculturation and White supremacist ideology. *American Psychologist, 74*(1), 143–55. https://doi.org/10.1037/amp0000368.

Lopez Mercado, D., Rivera-González, A. C., Stimpson, J. P., Langellier, B. A., et al. (2023). Undocumented Latino immigrants and the Latino health paradox. *American Journal of Preventive Medicine, 65*(2), 296–306. https://doi.org/10.1016/j.amepre.2023.02.010.

Lugones, M. (1987). Playfulness, "World"—travelling, and loving perception. *Hypatia, 2*(2), 3–19. www.jstor.org/stable/3810013.

Mossakowski, K. N. (2003). Coping with perceived discrimination: Does ethnic identity protect mental health? *Journal of Health and Social Behavior, 44*(3), 318–331. https://doi.org/10.2307/1519782.

Nava, G. (Director). (1997). *Selena* [Film]. Q-Productions.

Pérez, D. J., Fortuna, L., & Alegria, M. (2008). Prevalence and correlates of everyday discrimination among U.S. Latinos. *Journal of Community Psychology, 36*(4), 421–433. https://doi.org/10.1002/jcop.20221.

Sabina, C., Perez, G., Cuevas, C. A., & Farrell, A. (2023). Which Latinos experience bias victimization? An examination of acculturation, immigrant status, and socio-economic status. *Journal of Interpersonal Violence, 38*(17–18), 9898–9922. https://doi.org/10.1177/08862605231169775.

Smokowski, P. R., Rose, R. A., & Bacallao, M. (2010). Influence of risk factors and cultural assets on Latino adolescents' trajectories of self-esteem and internalizing symptoms. *Child Psychiatry and Human Development, 41*(2), 133–155. https://doi.org/10.1007/s10578-009-0157-6.

Substance Abuse and Mental Health Services Administration. (2014). *A Treatment Improvement Protocol: Improving Cultural Competence. TIP 59.* U.S. Department of Health and Human Services. www.ncbi.nlm.nih.gov/books/NBK248428/pdf/Bookshelf_NBK248428.pdf.

Sue, S. & Chu, J. Y. (2003). The mental health of ethnic minority groups: challenges posed by the Supplement to the Surgeon General's Report on Mental Health. *Culture, Medicine and Psychiatry, 27*(4), 447–465. https://doi.org/10.1023/B:MEDI.0000005483.80655.15.

Thornhill, C. W., Castillo, L. G., Piña-Watson, B., Manzo, G., & Cano, M. Á. (2022). Mental health among Latinx emerging adults: Examining the role of familial accusations of assimilation and ethnic identity. *Journal of Clinical Psychology, 78*(5), 892–912. https://doi.org/10.1002/jclp.23271.

Torres, L. (2010). Predicting levels of Latino depression: Acculturation, acculturative stress, and coping. *Cultural Diversity and Ethnic Minority Psychology, 16*(2), 256–263. https://doi.org/10.1037/a0017357.

Virupaksha, H. G., Kumar, A., & Nirmala, B. P. (2014). Migration and mental health: An interface. *Journal of Natural Science, Biology, and Medicine, 5*(2), 233–239. https://doi.org/10.4103/0976-9668.136141.

Yoon, E., Chang, C. T., Kim, S., Clawson, A., *et al.* (2013). A meta-analysis of acculturation/enculturation and mental health. *Journal of Counseling Psychology, 60*(1), 15–30. https://doi.org/10.1037/a0030652.

Chapter 9: Finding Healthy Collectivism: Balance, Setting Boundaries, Managing Expectations, and Challenging Unhelpful Guilt

Flores Niemann, Y. (2004). Stereotypes of Chicanas and Chicanos: Impact on Family Functioning, Individual Expectations, Goals, and Behavior. In R. J. Velásquez, L. M. Arellano, & B. W. McNeill (eds), *The Handbook of Chicana/o Psychology and Mental Health.* Lawrence Erlbaum Associates Publishers. https://doi.org/10.4324/9781410610911.

Green, R.-J. & Werner, P. D. (1996). Intrusiveness and closeness-caregiving: Rethinking the concept of family "enmeshment." *Family Process, 35*(2), 115–136. https://doi.org/10.1111/j.1545-5300.1996.00115.x.

Hemphill, P. [@prentishemphill]. (2021, April 5). *Boundaries are the distance at which I can love you and me simultaneously* [Photograph]. Instagram. www.instagram.com/p/CNSzFO1A21C/?hl=en.

Tawwab, N. G. (2021). *Set Boundaries, Find Peace: A Guide to Reclaiming Yourself.* Tarcher-Perigee, an imprint of Penguin Random House.

Chapter 10: Freeing Ourselves from the Colonization of Gender

Adames, H. Y. & Chavez-Dueñas, N. Y. (2017). *Cultural Foundations and Interventions in Latino/A Mental Health: History, Theory, and Within-Group Differences.* Routledge.

Allen, P. G. (1992). *The Sacred Hoop: Recovering the Feminine in American Indian Traditions* (first edition). Open Road Integrated Media, Inc.

Barnard, A. J. & Spencer, J. (1996). *Encyclopedia of Social and Cultural Anthropology*. Routledge.

Bonfil Batalla, G. (1996). *México Profundo: Reclaiming a Civilization*. University of Texas Press.

Boudreau, S. (n.d.). *Beyond just XX or XY: The complexities of biological sex*. Visiblebody. com. www.visiblebody.com/blog/beyond-just-xx-or-xy-the-complexities-of-biological-sex.

Burman, A. (2011). *Chachawarmi*: Silence and rival voices on decolonisation and gender politics in Andean Bolivia. *Journal of Latin American Studies, 43*(1), 65–91. https://doi.org/10.1017/S0022216X10001793.

Butler, J. (1988). Performative acts and gender constitution: An essay in phenomenology and feminist theory. *Theatre Journal, 40*(4), 519–531. https://doi.org/10.2307/3207893.

Fragoso, J. M. & Kashubeck, S. (2000). Machismo, gender role conflict, and mental health in Mexican American men. *Psychology of Men & Masculinity, 1*(2), 87–97. https://doi.org/10.1037/1524-9220.1.2.87.

Gabbatt, A. (2015, June 16). *Donald Trump's tirade on Mexico's "drugs and rapists" outrages US Latinos*. The Guardian. https://theguardian.com/us-news/2015/jun/16/donald-trump-mexico-presidential-speech-latino-hispanic.

Harvey, D., Smart, J., & Panero, J. (n.d.). *La Malinche, Hernán Cortés's translator and so much more*. The National Endowment for the Humanities. www.neh.gov/article/la-malinche-hernan-cortess-translator-and-so-much-more.

Horswell, M. (2006). *Decolonizing the Sodomite: Queer Tropes of Sexuality in Colonial Andean Culture*. University of Texas Press.

Jaquette, J. S. (1973). Women in revolutionary movements in Latin America. *Journal of Marriage and Family, 35*(2), 344–354. https://doi.org/10.2307/350664.

Jezzini, A. T. (2013). Acculturation, marianismo, gender role, and ambivalent sexism in predicting depression in Latinas. [Doctoral Dissertation, University of Denver]. Electronic Theses and Dissertations.

Kellogg, S. (2005). *Weaving the Past: A History of Latin America's Indigenous Women from the Prehispanic Period to the Present*. Oxford University Press.

Landers, J. (2013). Founding mothers: Female rebels in colonial New Granada and Spanish Florida. *Journal of African American History, 98*(1), 7–23. https://doi-org.csulb.idm.oclc.org/10.5323/jafriamerhist.98.1.0007.

Lugones, M. (2007). Heterosexualism and the colonial/modern gender system. *Hypatia, 22*(1), 186–209. www.jstor.org/stable/4640051.

Martínez, V. & Barajas, J. (2020, August 23). *The women of the Brown Berets—Las Adelitas de Aztlán—break free and form their own movement*. The Los Angeles Times. www.latimes.com/projects/chicano-moratorium/female-brown-berets-create-chicana-movement.

Mueller, A. S., Abrutyn, S., Pescosolido, B., & Diefendorf, S. (2021). The social roots of suicide: Theorizing how the external social world matters to suicide and suicide prevention. *Frontiers in Psychology, 12*, 621569. https://doi.org/10.3389/fpsyg.2021.621569.

Nieto, N. (2020). Mexican and Brazilian machismo: Cultural tolerance. *Journal of Comparative Studies, 13*(42), 104–126. https://doi.org/10.59893/jcs.13(42).006.

Nuñez, A., González, P., Talavera, G. A., Sanchez-Johnsen, L., *et al.* (2016). Machismo, marianismo, and negative cognitive-emotional factors: Findings from the Hispanic community health study/study of Latinos sociocultural ancillary study. *Journal of Latinx Psychology, 4*(4), 202–217. https://doi.org/10.1037/lat0000050.

Oyěwùmí, O. (1997). *The Invention of Women: Making an African Sense of Western Gender Discourses*. University of Minnesota Press.

Sigal, P. (2011). *The Flower and the Scorpion: Sexuality and Ritual in Early Nahua Culture*. Duke University Press. https://doi.org/10.2307/j.ctv1220pch.

Sousa, L. (2017). *The Woman who Turned into a Jaguar, and Other Narratives of Native Women in Archives of Colonial Mexico*. Stanford University Press.

Stern, S. J. (1995). *The Secret History of Gender: Women, Men, and Power in Late Colonial Mexico*. University of North Carolina Press.

Tello, J. (2008). El Hombre Noble Buscando Balance: The Noble Man Searching for Balance. In R. Carrillo & J. Tello (eds), *Family Violence and Men of Color: Healing the Wounded Male Spirit*. Springer Publishing Company.

The Trevor Project. (2023, October 12). *Report: Latinx LGBTQ young people face unique mental health challenges and disparities in suicide risk, attempts*. The Trevor Project. www.thetrevorproject.org/blog/report-latinx-lgbtq-young-people-face-unique-mental-health-challenges-and-disparities-in-suicide-risk-attempts.

Udo, E. M. (2020). The vitality of Yoruba culture in the Americas. *Ufahamu: A Journal of African Studies, 41*(2). https://doi.org/10.5070/f7412046833.

Valdez, L. A., Jaeger, E. C., Garcia, D. O., & Griffith, D. M. (2023). Breaking down machismo: Shifting definitions and embodiments of Latino manhood in middle-aged Latino men. *American Journal of Men's Health, 17*(5). https://doi.org/10.1177/15579883231195118.

Wagner, E. (n.d.). *Person: Emma Tenayuca*. National Park Service. www.nps.gov/people/emma-tenayuca.htm.

Webb, H. S. (2012). *Yanantin and Masintin in the Andean World Complementary Dualism in Modern Peru*. University of New Mexico Press.

Wolfson, S. Q. (2023, October 16). *Traitor, ghost, feminist icon: Reclaiming the stories of La Llorona*. The Los Angeles Times. www.latimes.com/delos/story/2023-10-16/la-llorona-mexico-latin-america-horror-folklore.

Chapter 11: Getting Out of Survival Mode and Back into the Body

Siegel, D. & Bryson, T. P. (2011). *The Whole-Brain Child: 12 Proven Strategies to Nurture Your Child's Developing Mind*. Delacorte Press.

Clapp, J. (2020). *Movement for Trauma Training Manual: Fall 2020*. Jane Clapp. www.janeclapp.com.

Dana, D. A. & Porges, S. W. (2018). *The Polyvagal Theory in Therapy: Engaging the Rhythm of Regulation*. W. W. Norton.

EMDR Consulting. (2020). *Integrating EMDR into Your Clinical Practice Intensive Training Manual*. EMDR Consulting.

Estés, C. P. (1995). *Women Who Run with the Wolves: Myths and Stories of the Wild Woman Archetype*. Ballantine Books.

Godek, D. & Freeman, A. M. (2022, September 26). *Physiology, Diving reflex*. www.ncbi.nlm.nih.gov/books/NBK538245.

Pattakos, A. (2010). *Prisoners of Our Thoughts: Viktor Frankl's Principles for Discovering Meaning in Life and Work* (second edition). Berrett-Koehler Publishers.

Porges, S. (2016). The Neurobiology of Trauma, Attachment, Self-Regulation & Emotions [Workshop presentation]. PESI.

Schwartz, A. (2018). Complex PTSD 2-day clinical workshop: A Comprehensive Approach to Accurately Assess and Effectively Treat Clients with Chronic, Repeated, and/or Developmental Trauma [Workshop presentation]. PESI.

Substance Abuse and Mental Health Services Administration. (2014). *SAMHSA's Concept of Trauma and Guidance for a Trauma-Informed Approach*. HHS Publication.

Substance Abuse and Mental Health Services Administration. (2014). *Trauma-Informed Care in Behavioral Health Services. Treatment Improvement Protocol (TIP) Series 57*. HHS Publication.

Walker, P. (2013). *Complex PTSD: From Surviving to Thriving*. Azure Coyote.

Walker, R. J. (2023). *Polyvagal Theory Chart of Trauma Response*. Southwest Trauma Training. www.swtraumatraining.com/recources.

Weathers, F. W., Blake, D. D., Schnurr, P. P., Kaloupek, D. G., Marx, B. P., & Keane, T. M. (2013). The Life Events Checklist for DSM-5 (LEC-5). Instrument available from the National Center for PTSD at www.ptsd.va.gov.

Chapter 12: Learning to Feel Our Feelings, Challenge Negative Belief Systems, and Process Our Trauma

Bolte Taylor, J. (2022). *Whole Brain Living: The Anatomy of Choice and the Four Characters that Drive Our Life*. Hay House.

Brach, T. (2019). *Radical Compassion: Learning to Love Yourself and Your World with the Practice of RAIN*. Viking Life.

Haines, S. (2019). *The Politics of Trauma: Somatics, Healing, and Social Justice*. North Atlantic Books.

Shapiro, F. (2012). *Getting Past Your Past: Take Control of Your Life with Self-Help Techniques from EMDR Therapy*. Rodale.

Siegel, D. & Bryson, T. P. (2011). *The Whole-Brain Child: 12 Proven Strategies to Nurture Your Child's Developing Mind*. Delacorte Press.

Chapter 13: *Hoy Semillas, Mañanas Flores*
(Today Seeds—Tomorrow Flowers)

Acosta, A. & Abarca, M. M. (2018). Buen Vivir: An Alternative Perspective from the Peoples of the Global South to the Crisis of capitalist modernity. In V. Satgar (ed.), *The Climate Crisis: South African and Global Democratic Eco-Socialist Alternatives* (pp.131–147). Wits University Press. https://doi.org/10.18772/22018020541.11.

Albó, X. (2018). *Suma Qamaña* or Living Well Together: A Contribution to Biocultural Conservation. In R. Rozzi, *et al.* (eds), *Biocultural Homogenization to Biocultural Conservation. Ecology and Ethics, vol 3*. Springer, Cham. https://doi.org/10.1007/978-3-319-99513-7_21.

Comas-Díaz, L. (2020). Liberation Psychotherapy. In L. Comas-Díaz & E. Torres Rivera (eds), *Liberation Psychology: Theory, Method, Practice, and Social Justice* (pp.169–185). American Psychological Association.

Isasi-Diaz, A. M. (2004*). En la Lucha/In the Struggle: Elaborating a Mujerista Theology*. Fortress Press.

Marcos, S. (2002). *Our word is our weapon*. https://theanarchistlibrary.org/library/subcomandante-marcos-our-word-is-our-weapon.

Parker, P. (1983). Revolution: It's Not Neat or Pretty or Quick. In C. Moraga & G. Anzaldua, *This Bridge Called My Back: Writings by Radical Women of Colour* (second edition) (pp.238–242). Kitchen Table Press.

Telégrafo, E. (2013, April 7). *¿Qué es el Sumak Kawsay?* El Telégrafo. www.eltelegrafo.com.ec/noticias/columnistas/1/que-es-el-sumak-kawsay.

Appendix

Bishop, M. & Vargas, C. (2014, May 2). *The Invention of Hispanics*. NPR. www.latinousa.org/2014/05/02/invention-hispanics.

Ramos, P. (2020). *Finding Latinx: In Search of the Voices Redefining Latino Identity*. Vintage Books, a division of Penguin Random House LLC.

Simón, Y. (2023, September 25). *Latino, Hispanic, Latinx, Chicano: The history behind the terms*. History. www.history.com/news/hispanic-latino-latinx-chicano-background.

Zong, J. (2022, October 26). *A mosaic, not a monolith: A profile of the U.S. Latino population, 2000–2020*. UCLA Latino Policy & Politics Institute. https://latino.ucla.edu/research/latino-population-2000-2020.

Index

accountability in
    culture 110–12
acculturation 136–40,
    143–4, 145
Acuña, Elisa 180
Adames, Hector Y. 171
aesthetics
    and white
        supremacy 79
African slavery
    abolition of 52
    in Latin America and
        Caribbean 42–6
Afro-Latinxs
    and colorism 57, 58
    and construction of
        racial groups 56
    in United States 59
Aguilar, Sofía 58
Alexander VI, Pope 31
Allen, Paula Gunn 169
Allende, Salvador 123
Alvarado, Pedro de 35
Amaru, Cecilia Tupac 180
American Psychiatric
    Association (APA) 84
ancestral resources 112–15
Andean civilizations
    conquest of 34–7
    cultures of 27–30
    gender in 168–9
    pre-colonial
        populations 37
Anzaldua, Gloria 27, 93
Arawaks 33
Arce, Julissa 135
Arellano, Juan
    Estevan 108

Argentina
    construction of racial
        groups in 54, 55
    neoliberalism in 130
    United States
        interventions
        in 124
assimilation 145–9
Atahualpa 36
automatic stress
    responses
    190–200, 204–9
ayllus 29
Aymara civilization
    28, 168–9, 229
Aztec civilization see
    Mexica civilization

Bachelet, Michelle 130
Bacio, Guadalupe 143
Bahamas 3
balance and harmony 106
Baldwin, James 67
Banaji, Mahzarin R. 64
Barajas, Clara 142
Batalla, Guillermo
    Bonfil 168
bell hooks 80
Beyond Slavery: The
    Multilayered Legacy
    of Africans in Latin
    America and the
    Caribbean (Davis) 56
binary thinking
    and white supremacy
    71–3
Black in Latin America
    (Gates) 56

blood quantum 97
Bolivia 54, 124, 130, 229
Bolte Taylor, Jill 212
boundaries
    emotional 157
    and expectation
        management
        158–60
    in families 153–5
    intellectual 155–6
    material 157–8
    physical 155
    sexual 156
    time 157
Bracero program 131
Brave Heart, Maria Yellow
    Horse 18, 86, 87, 92
Brazil
    African slavery in
        43, 44, 52
    colonization in 39, 40
    construction of racial
        groups in 54, 56
    forest-dwelling
        groups in 33
    neoliberalism in 130
    Portuguese interest
        in 31–2
    United States
        interventions
        in 124
breath work 25–6, 204
Broken Spears, The: The
    Aztec Account of the
    Conquest of Mexico
    (Leon-Portilla) 34, 36
Brown v Board of
    Education 61, 89

buen vivir 228-32
Bukele, Nayib 123
Butler, Judith 166

Cáceres, Berta 98
Calzada, Esther 145
capitalism
and neoliberalism
125-30
and white supremacy
73-5
Caribbean
African slavery in 42-6
colonialization
of 38-42
conquest of 33
pre-colonial
populations 33, 37
Caribs 33
Castañeda, Heidie 118
Cervantes, Andrea
Gómez 122
Chavez-Dueñas,
Nayeli Y. 171
Chicano movement 96
Chile 54, 123-4, 130
Chu, June 143
Cihuacoati 178
Clinton, Bill 126-7
Coatsworth, John 119
collective trauma see
historical trauma
collectivism
and boundaries 153-8
and enmeshment
153-5
and expectation
management
158-60
and familism 104-5,
109-10, 150-5
guilt in 160-2
colorism 57-9
Columbus, Christopher
30, 33
compadrazgo 150-1
Cortés, Hernán 36, 175-6
Cosmic Race, The
(Vasconcelos) 53-4
cosmovision 107
Costa Rica 54
Coyolxauhqui
imperative 93
criollo peoples 49, 52-3
Cuba
African slavery in 44-5

construction of racial
groups in 52, 56
United States
interventions
in 124
Cuevas, C.A. 111
culture
accountability
in 110-12
and acculturation
136-40, 143-4, 145
ancestral resources
for 112-15
and assimilation 145-9
and generational
trauma 20-1
indigenous influences
on Latinx
culture 104-9
and language
loss 140-2
of Mesoamerican
and Andean
civilizations 27-30
negative expressions
of 109-10
strength in 100-2
and transculturation
102-4

Davis, Darién J. 56
DeGruy, Joy 92
Devos, Thierry 64
Diagnostic and Statistical
Manual of Mental
Disorders (DSM)
(APA) 84, 85
Diego, Juan 176-7
Dismantling Racism 80
displacement from
land 95-6
dominance
and white supremacy
68-9
Dominican Republic 124
Dunbar-Ortiz,
Roxanne 98
Duran, Bonnie 91
Duran, Eduardo 91

Ecuador 55, 124, 229
Eisenhower, Dwight
D. 120
El Salvador 121-3
Ellison, C.G. 116

emotional regulation
210-11
emotions
boundaries for 157
and emotional
regulation 210-11
and negative beliefs
215-17
and positive belief
strengthening
217-19
understanding
of 211-14
En la Lucha/In the Struggle
(Isasi-Díaz) 227
encomienda system 39
enfermedad del alma (soul
wounds) 91-3, 101
Engel, Patricia 13
enmeshment 153-5
Estés, Clarissa Pinkola 187
eugenic sterilization 89
Evans-Campbell,
Teresa 92
expectation management
158-60
Eye Movement and
Desensitization
and Reprocessing
(EMDR) 218

Failed (Weisbrot) 126
familismo/familism
balancing with
self 162-4
and collectivism 150-5
indigenous influence
on 104-5
negative aspects
of 109-10
Family Violence and Men
of Color: Healing
the Wounded Male
Spirit (Tello) 171
Farah, Douglas 120
Feminist Theory: From
Margin to Center
(hooks) 80
Fernandez, Alberto 54
Ferdinand II, King 30
fight response 191,
192, 195-6, 197,
198, 199, 200
flight response 191,
192, 193-5, 197,
197, 198, 199, 200

Flower and the Scorpion, The (Sigal) 182
For Brown Girls with Sharp Edges and Tender Hearts: A Love Letter to Women of Color (Rodríguez) 63
Frankl, Viktor 190
Franzini, L. 142
freeze response 191, 192, 196, 197, 198, 199, 200, 206–8
Freire, Paulo 23, 70

Garcia, Denia 58–9
Gates, Henry Louis Jr 56
Geiger, Gabriella 145
gender
    archetypes of femininity 175–8
    and colonisation 169–70
    gender binary 165–6
    and machismo 166, 170–4
    and marianismo 166, 174–81
    and masculinity 170–4
    performance of 166–7
    in pre-colonial societies 167–9, 181–2
    queer people 181–5
    trans people 181–5
generational trauma
    and culture 20–1
    definition of 19–20
Gortari, Carlos Salinas de 127
grief 99–100
Guatemala
    construction of racial groups in 55
    United States intervention in 120–1
guilt 160–2
gun violence 90–1

Haiti 124
Handbook of Chicana/o Psychology and Mental Health, The (Velásquez *et al.*) 22

healing
    and emotional regulation 210–11
    facing trauma 219–20
    intentional safety 202–3
    and negative beliefs 215–17
    and positive belief strengthening 217–19
    as process 186–90
    and societal change 226–8
    soothing the nervous system 200–1
    starting 17–17
    testimonio writing 220–5
    tools for automatic stress response 204–9
health outcomes 142–5
Heilemann, Marysue 143
Hemmings, Betty 51
Hemmings, Sally 51
Hernández, Tanya Katerí 56
Hill, Megan Minoka 97
Hispanics as category 234–5
historical trauma
    definition of 18
    in Latinx community 18
    naming of 86–7
    and mental health issues 84–6
    and sense of loss 95–100
    and soul wounds 91–3
Honduras 124
hooks, bell 80
Huáscar 35
humildad/humility 105

Immigration and Customs Enforcement (ICE) 89, 90, 132
Indian in Latin American History, The (Kicza) 37
indigeneity 96–8
indigenous influences on Latinx culture 104–9
Indigenous Peoples' History of the United States, An (Dunbar-Ortiz) 98

individual trauma
    definition of 20
individualism
    and white supremacy 75–7
Inka civilization 28, 32, 35–6
intellectual boundaries 155–6
intentional safety 202–3
International Monetary Fund (IMF) 125, 126
Institute of Chicana/o/x Psychology 101
Invention of Women, The: Making an African Sense of Western Gender Discourses (Oyěwùmí) 167
Isabella I, Queen 30, 31
Isasi-Díaz, Ada María 227
Izadi, E. 64

Jefferson, Thomas 51
Johnson, Michelle 80
Juana 179–80

Katz, Judith H. 65
Kicza, John 37
Koch, Alexander 37

La Guera (Moraga) 57
La Llorona (suffering woman archetype) 177–8
La Malinche (traitor archetype) 175–6
La Virgen (perfect woman archetype) 176–7
Landa, Diego de 27
language loss 140–2
Las Adelitas de Aztlán 180
Las Castas paintings 51
Latin America
    African slavery in 42–6
    colonialization of 38–42
    colorism in 57–9
    conquest of 34–7
    construction of racial groups in 48–56
    gender in pre-colonial 168–9

Latin America *cont.*
  migration to United
    States 119–25,
    129–33
  neoliberal policies
    in 125–6, 130
  pre-colonial
    cultures 27–30
  pre-colonial
    populations 37
  United States
    interventions
    in 119–25
Latinx people
  accountability
    in 110–12
  acculturation 136–40,
    143–4, 145
  and Afro-Latinxs
    56, 57, 58, 59
  and assimilation 145–9
  and colorism 57–9
  as description 13–15
  gender constructs
    in 166
  health outcomes
    of 142–5
  historical trauma
    in 18, 87–91
  indigenous influences
    on 104–9
  and language
    loss 140–2
  and machismo 170–4
  and marianismo 174–81
  and mental health
    issues 85–6
  and migration
    narratives
    116–17, 132
  origins of term 14
  population in United
    States 13, 87,
    118–19
  queer and trans
    people 181–5
  and sense of loss
    95–100
  and soul wounds
    91–3, 101
  and systems of
    oppression 82
  and transculturation
    102–3
  and white supremacy
    66–7

Lau, Anna 143
Lavoe, Hector 104
Leal, D.L. 116
Leon-Portilla, Miguel 34
liberation
  and buen vivir 228–32
  definition of 20
  need for solidarity
    98–9
  and societal change
    226–8
*Light in the Dark/Luz en lo
  Oscuro* (Anzaldúa) 93
Liu, William Ming 147
Lopez, Alan Pelaez 14
loss, sense of 95–100
Lugones, María 148
lynchings 88–9

machismo 166, 170–4
Malintzin 175–6
Marcos, Subcomandante
  230–1
marianismo 166, 174–81
Martín-Baró, Ignacio 122
material boundaries
  157–8
Maya civilization 27, 28,
  32, 54, 120, 176, 229
Mays, Vickie 143
Menakem, Resmaa 20–1
Mendez v. Westminster
  61
Menjívar, Cecilia 122
mental health issues
  and historical
    trauma 84–6
  as medical model 84–5
Mesoamerican
  civilizations
  conquest of 34–7
  cultures of 27–30
  gender in 168, 181–2
  pre-colonial
    populations 37
mestizaje system 49,
  53–6, 58–9
mestizo peoples 49,
  50, 53, 54, 55, 176
Mexica civilization 28,
  32, 34, 35, 36, 171
Mexican-American war
  (1846–48) 87, 88
Mexico
  construction of racial
    groups in 54, 55

migration to United
  States 87–8,
  129–30, 131
  and North American
    Free Trade
    Agreement
    (NAFTA) 126–30
*México Profundo:
  Reclaiming a
  Civilization*
  (Batalla) 168
migration
  from Latin America
    119–25, 129–33
  stories of 116–18
  United States
    policies 130–4
  as universal
    experience 118
Minas Gerais 40
mita system 39, 42–3
Montezuma 35
Moraga, Cherríe 57
Morales, Eva 130
Morrison, Toni 64
Mossakowski, Krysia 145
My Grandmother's Hands
  (Menakem) 20–1

National Council of La
  Raza (NCLR) 234–5
*Native American
  Postcolonial Psychology*
  (Duran & Duran) 91
negative beliefs 215–17
neoliberalism 125–30
nervous system
  soothing 200–1
neuroception 191
*New World of Gold and
  Silver, A* (TePaske) 41
Nicaragua 124
Nixon, Richard 234
Noe-Bustamante, Luis 57
North American Free
  Trade Agreement
  (NAFTA) 126–30

objectivity
  and white supremacy
    70–1
Office of Homeland
  Security Statistics
  132
Olmec civilization 28

"On Naming Ourselves,
Or When I was a
Spic" (Engel) 13
Orozco, José Clemente 54
Oyěwùmí, Oyèrónkè 167

Panama 124
Paraguay 124
Pavon, José María
Morelos y 52
Pedagogy of the Oppressed
(Freire) 23
perfectionism
and white supremacy
67–8
person-in-environment
perspective 22
personalismo 106–7
Peru
colonization in 40
construction of racial
groups in 55
Pew Research Center
57, 59, 141, 235
physical boundaries 155
Pinochet, Augusto 123–4
Pizarro, Fransisco 36
Polo, Marco 30
Porges, Stephen 191
Portuguese colonialism
conquests of 34–7
and gender 169–70
reasons for 31–2
positive belief
strengthening 217–19
Post Traumatic Slave
Syndrome (DeGruy)
92
Postero, Nancy Grey 55
Potosí 40, 41
praxis 23, 122, 187,
211, 226, 227
Prisoners of Our
Thoughts: Viktor
Frankl's Principles
for Discovering
Meaning in Life and
Work (Frankl) 190
Project on Ethnicity
and Race in Latin
America 56
Protestant Work Ethic 75
Public Citizen 128
Puerto Rico 89
Purchasing Whiteness
(Twinam) 50

qariwarmi 181
quality of life
and white supremacy
73–5
Quechua civilization 28
queer people 181–5
querencia 108–9
Quesada, Kayla
Popuchet 82
quilombos communities 45

Racial Innocence:
Unmasking Latino
Anti-Black Bias and the
Struggle for Equality
(Hernández) 56
Ramírez III, Manuel 22
Re-indigenizing 101
Reagan, Ronald 127
Reflective Democracy
Campaign 60–1
repatriation drives 89–90
responsibilidad/
responsibility 105
right to comfort
and white supremacy
77–8
Rivera, Diego 54
Rivera, Sylvia 180
Rodríguez, Prisca
Dorcas Mojica 63

Sabina, Chiara 111, 144
Sacred Hoop, The:
Recovering the Feminine
in American Indian
Traditions (Allen) 169
Secret History of Gender,
The: Women, Men, and
Power in Late Colonial
Mexico (Stern) 170
segregation 89
Selena (film) 135
sexual boundaries 156
Shin, H. 116
Siegel, Dan 200, 213
Sigal, Pete 182
Silva Luiz Inácio da
"Lula" 130
simpatia 106–7, 109–10
Siqueiros, David
Alfaro 54
slavery see African slavery
Smokowski, Paul 143
Sotero, Michelle 18

soul wounds 91–3, 101
Spanish colonialism
conquests of 34–7
and gender 169–70
reasons of 30–1
spirituality 107–8
Stern, Steve 170
Struggle for Indigenous
Rights in Latin
America (Postero
and Zamosc) 55
Substance Abuse
and Mental
Health Services
Administration
(SAMHSA) 18
Sue, Stanley 143
systems of oppression
80–3

Taino peoples 33, 96
Tecum 35
Telles, Edward 58–9
Tello, Jerry 171
Tenayuca, Emma 180
Tenochtitlán 32, 34, 179
TePaske, John 41
testimonio writing 220–5
Thornhill, Carly 138
time boundaries 157
Toltec civilization 28
Tonantzin 176–7
trans people 181–5
transculturation 102–4
trauma
automatic stress
responses to
190–200
and culture 20–1
definition of 18
and emotional
regulation 210–11
facing 219–20
and healing process
186–90
intentional safety
202–3
and negative beliefs
215–17
and positive belief
strengthening
217–19
soothing the nervous
system 200–1
testimonio writing
220–5

trauma *cont.*
tools for automatic
stress response
204–9
Trevor Project 183
Trump, Donald 170
Tupi people 34, 43
Twinam, Ann 50

U.S. Government
Accountability
Office 110
UnidosUS 75, 235
United Nations
Declaration on the
Rights of Indigenous
Peoples 97
United States
colorism in 57, 59
construction of racial
groups in 59–61
and Hispanics as
category 234–5
interventions in Latin
America 119–25
Latin American
migration to
119–25, 129–33
Latinx population
in 13, 87, 118–19
migration narratives in
116–17, 132, 133–4
migration policies
130–3
systems of oppression
in 80

white supremacy in
60–1, 64–80
*Universal Declaration of
the Rights of Mother
Earth* (World People's
Conference on
Climate Change
and the Rights of
Mother Earth) 107
Uruguay 54

Vasconcelos, José 53–4
Velásquez, R.J. 22
Venezuela 124
Volkan, Vamik 19

Wall Street (film) 73
Washington, George 60
Washington Consensus
125–6
Wayles, John 51
Weisbrot, Mark 126
Whitbeck, Les B. 92
white supremacy
aesthetics in 79
and assimilation
146–8
binary thinking in
71–3
capitalism in 73–5
dominance in 68–9
individualism in 75–7
objectivity in 70–1
perfectionism in
67–8

quality of life in 73–5
qualities of 67–79
right to comfort
in 77–8
in United States
60–1, 64–80
Wills, C. 111
Wilson, Michael 127
Window of Tolerance
200–1
*Women Who Run with
the Wolves* (Estés)
187
Worden, J. William 99
World Bank 125
World People's
Conference on
Climate Change
and the Rights of
Mother Earth 107

Yehuda, Rachel 19
Yoon, Eunju 143
*You Sound Like a White
Girl* (Arce) 135

Zamarripa, Manuel 101
Zamosc, Leon 55
Zapata, Emiliano 180
Zapatista Army of
National Liberation
(EZLN) 128, 180
Zapotec civilization 28
Ziwe 30